The Crisis in
Clinical Research

THE CRISIS IN CLINICAL RESEARCH

Overcoming Institutional Obstacles

EDWARD H. AHRENS, JR.

New York   Oxford
OXFORD UNIVERSITY PRESS
1992

Oxford University Press

Oxford   New York   Toronto
Delhi   Bombay   Calcutta   Madras   Karachi
Petaling Jaya   Singapore   Hong Kong   Tokyo
Nairobi   Dar es Salaam   Cape Town
Melbourne   Auckland

and associated companies in
Berlin   Ibadan

Copyright © 1992 by Oxford University Press, Inc.

Published by Oxford University Press, Inc.,
200 Madison Avenue, New York, New York 10016

Oxford is a registered trademark of Oxford University Press

Library of Congress Cataloging-in-Publication Data
Ahrens, Edward H., 1915-
The crisis in clinical research : overcoming
institutional obstacles / Edward H. Ahrens, Jr.
p. cm.   Includes bibliographical references and index.
ISBN 0-19-505156-4
1. National Institutes of Health (U.S.) 2.
Federal aid to medical research—United States.
3. Medical policy—United States.
I. Title. [DNLM: 1. National Institutes of Health (U.S.).
2. Health Planning—United States.
3. Medicine—United States.
4. Research—United States.   CP W 20.5 A287c]
RA11.D6A37   1992   610′.72073—dc20
DNLM/DLC   for Library of Congress
91-32064

9 8 7 6 5 4 3 2 1

Printed in the United States of America
on acid-free paper

Preface

I retired from an active career in clinical research in 1985, after 40 years spent exploring a number of key questions in human biology through studies on whole human beings. Toward the end of that long period, I recognized a marked shift in the attitudes of medical scientists toward the goals of clinical research and in their perceptions of the roles they should play in its pursuit. A troubling question became inescapable: Is the study of whole human beings—which has proceeded so fruitfully for more than five decades—no longer essential? Has that painstaking endeavor become so outmoded by the advent of speedier and more elegant modern technologies of molecular biology that the many remaining problems of human disease will be solved solely at the bench rather than at the bedside?

These concerns led me to spend the last five years in fact finding and data gathering on this issue, as a result of which I have gained irrefutable evidence that the study of whole humans is indeed languishing today. But, in addition, that evidence is strongly persuasive that this kind of research is absolutely essential in furthering the study of human health and disease. This book will present the reasons for reaching these two conclusions.

In the course of this undertaking, I came to realize that far more than the study of human biology is in jeopardy in today's medical world: It appears that American medicine *as a whole* is in trouble. It became clear to me that the three traditional missions of U.S. medical schools—teaching medical students, providing service to patients, and performing research at the frontier of knowledge—are now seriously out of balance. Indeed, these three functions of modern medical schools are so intimately intertwined that problems in one arena have serious repercussions for all three. So, although the main emphasis of this book is directed at the future outlook for clinical research, my story would be incomplete and one-sided if I failed to remind the reader at every appropriate stage that research is only one element—the exploring element—in the activities of medical schools that also must teach and render services to the public.

To begin, we will look at the broad picture of American medicine—doctors and medical schools, and the institutional settings in which research takes place. Clinical research will be carefully categorized into the several kinds of research activities taking place under this broad umbrella term; and the current status and future outlook for each of these activities will be discussed. Then the role of research in relation to service and education in academic health centers will be carefully weighed as we explore the commonly held perception that American medicine as a whole is seriously troubled, for any remedies applied to the problems of research will be futile unless the far broader issues are addressed and understood. The most compelling question, of course, is whether academic physicians can any longer do justice to the three roles they play in a medical center when each of the three—teaching, service, and research—is so time-consuming.

In 1910, Abraham Flexner published a lengthy report that riveted the attention of educators generally and the medical profession in particular on the deficiencies of medical education in the United States and Canada, a report that led to a series of reforms, the effects of which are felt right up to the present. Flexner's detailed analysis of each of the 155 North American medical schools was a damning description of their sad state at the turn of the century: Most of these schools were run for profit, and Flexner urged that all but 31 of them be abolished. His report was an eloquent plea for abandoning the profit motive and forging closer ties between universities and those medical schools that were willing to modernize by bringing science into medicine. These changes have been largely completed, and now is an appropriate time to examine the consequences.

Flexner appealed for sweeping reforms in a decadent educational system. The book now in hand points not at decadence but at imbalances. My study grew out of personal pride in the profession of medicine, and out of my admiration for all that has been achieved during this century in new understandings of health and disease. Nevertheless, I feel deep concern for its future: I intend to present the evidence underlying that concern in order to justify consideration of a number of recommendations aimed at correcting those imbalances.

New York   E.H.A., Jr.
February 1991

Acknowledgment

It is my pleasure to take this opportunity to thank the many friends, old and new, who have been so helpful to me over the last six years in my desire to reach a deeper understanding of the many aspects of the situations addressed in this book—educational, economic, political and sociological, as well as scientific. The reference list and the index contain many of the names of experts on whom I have leaned for advice; further than this, I have intentionally omitted references to many important contributors in the interest of keeping the text as lean and pointed as possible. To the literally hundreds of individuals with whom I have had enormously informative conversations, I can only say, "Thank you." But there are still others, named below, who have been so eminently helpful that I cannot fail to pay them the special courtesy of naming them.

My fact-finding and impression-gathering began in 1985 with a series of four 2-day meetings here at the Rockefeller University over a 4-month period, each attended by a different half-dozen articulators from various walks of life, all informed about clinical research in some way. Alphabetically listed they were:

Beeson, Paul B.	Mustard, J. Fraser
Bloom, Floyd E.	Oates, John A.
Capron, Alexander M.	Petersdorf, Robert G.
Chalmers, Thomas C.	Relman, Arnold S.
Cole, Jonathan	Ross, Richard S.
Dunlop, John T.	Rubinstein, Arthur
Gross, Jerome	Schoen, Donald A.
Hamburg, David	Stead, Eugene A., Jr.
Kennedy, Eugene P.	Thier, Samuel O.
Kern, Fred J.	White, Raymond C.
Kipnis, David M.	Wilson, Jean D.
Krugman, Saul	Wyngaarden, James B.
Littlefield, John W.	

These meetings were free-wheeling discussions on four major aspects of clinical research—with no prepared papers or set pieces. They were recorded and transcribed for my use only. These sessions were tremendously helpful in opening my eyes and ears to many issues I had not previously recognized, and in setting my path of inquiry for the next four years before I sat down to organize what I had learned.

I am particularly indebted to the 73 Program Directors of the GCRCs who gave so generously of their time and wisdom. A few were *more* than supportive and went the "extra mile": Robert G. Campbell, Robert E. Canfield, John W. Ensinck, Charles Y.C. Pak, Seymour Reichlin, Gary L. Robertson, R. Paul Robertson, and Michael O. Thorner. And for a similar kind of assistance I must express my gratitude to the (then) 12 NIH Institutes' Clinical Directors from whom I learned much about the inner workings of bedside research at the NIH.

For special tasks of data collection I acknowledge my deep indebtedness to Paul Jolly (AAMC), Gene Roback (AMA), Ruth Bulger (IOM), and in various offices of the NIH: John L. Decker, Jerome G. Green, Robert E. Moore, Lucille Nierzwicki, James F. O'Donnell, and Charles R. Sherman. And for many kinds of morale-boosting, direction-setting, and personal introductions, I am pleased to recognize Clarence L. Barnhart, Carleton B. Chapman, Jonathan Cole, John W. Gardner, Ann Harris, William N. Kelley, Richard L. Landau, Martha de Marre, Carol Moberg, Garrison Rapmund, Darwin Stapleton, Humphrey Taylor, Alan Simpson, and Richard F. Snow: each will recognize the special help given me so generously.

Finally, I thank two officers of this University—Joshua Lederberg, President, and David Lyons, Vice-President and Treasurer—who understood the importance of my undertaking and underwrote all its expenses for these six years. And special thanks to Rachael Kolb of this University, without whose computer-wisdom I would still be swimming in a sea of data.

Contents

The Crisis in
Clinical Research

1

Medicine in Trouble: General Perceptions

The perception that American medicine is in trouble has been growing for many years, with increasingly serious concerns being expressed by its many participants: practicing physicians (92% of American doctors) and those who teach (the other 8%); the administrators who supervise the provision of medical services in more than 5,000 hospitals; and by the public itself.

The troubles are partly economic. It costs more and more to provide optimal care, even though the U.S. population is becoming increasingly healthy. The repayment of skyrocketing medical care costs is becoming increasingly complex and bewildering, not only for the 85% of the public who are insured, but also for the insurers (including the Medicare system) that must cope with the rising costs of sophisticated new medical technologies. Hospitals are struggling to bridge the gap between their expenditures and the fixed charges allowed by the federal government for more than 400 different diseases, conditions and procedures. In addition, the cost of medical school education has become a serious burden on students. Finally, the costs of biomedical research (both direct and indirect) have escalated to such a degree that new researchers are being starved out.

Added to these economic woes are certain dispiriting changes in the delivery system itself as doctors leave solo practice and accept the loss of autonomy inherent in salaried employment, and as the profession increasingly comes to regard its activities as a highly specialized trade. For today's patients, an office visit is not very different from a visit to the local automobile mechanic—in both cases to fix a condition that the owner lacks the skill to fix himself.

What a paradox it is that such serious concerns have grown over the same decades in which so many stunning achievements have occurred in medical science, in the practice of medicine, and in the realization of important gains in the health of the public. These include a steady increase in life expectancy as infant and child mortality rates have decreased; substantial decreases in death due to stroke, heart attack, and cancer; the abolition of smallpox worldwide and the near-disappearance of poliomyelitis in the industrialized countries; technical innovations that have led to speedier, more exact, and less invasive diagnostic methods; and a steadily rising ratio of doctors and paramedical personnel to total population, with striking increases of women and minorities in the profession.

This chapter will deal with the general perception that American medicine is in deep trouble. Proceeding from the general to the particular, I will look first at the viewpoints of the public, then those of institutional leaders in medicine, and finally, the concerns of medical academics and researchers.

THE SOCIETAL EXPECTATIONS GAP

Even as late as the 1960s, the public had come to expect all good things from medicine: a long and happy life; freedom from the major killers (heart disease, cancer, and stroke); and the benefits of preventive medicine proffered at an affordable cost by skilled practitioners who were unhurried, gracious, reassuring, caring, and, above all, available. In Colloton's (1989) words, this was "the nature of academic medicine's long-standing covenant with society," having "its origins in trust" and "based on the premise that academic medicine's unique programs and commitments were substantial societal contributions, and thus justified generous support and the privilege of self-regulation." This was the social contract between medicine and the public—health and happiness at low cost.

The rise in public expectations of medicine came partly from the medical triumphs heralded as breakthroughs in the press almost daily but also from the general belief that health is a right to which everyone is entitled. But today, "the societal trust underlying our long-standing covenant is rapidly giving way to the clarion call for accountability and shared decision-making on many fronts" (Colloton, 1989).

In 1960 C. P. Snow delivered a series of lectures titled *The Two Cultures,* in which he described the gulf that developed between scientists and non-scientists. (Snow was a man with a foot in each camp, a physical scientist who was also a talented writer of fiction.) Speaking of scientists and non-scientists (and he was not thinking narrowly of science vs. humanism), he noted: "between the two a gulf of mutual incomprehension—sometimes hostility and dislike, but most of all, lack of understanding."

Despite the vast improvements that science writers have made in interpreting science to the public over the last 50 years, I believe that, while public understanding of science today may be broader, it is more superficial than ever before, becoming even anti-intellectual. True, more members of the general public have become accustomed to the terminologies of cosmology, physics, ecology, and biology than ever before, but the mental effort spent in reading about science is now spread more thinly over a broader landscape. The same people who are sufficiently educated to make their way in business, the law, politics, and religion seem to excuse their scientific illiteracy by saying that science has become too complicated to be understood and appreciated by non-scientists. How many intelligent laymen have any real understanding of the functions of their own bodies—pulse, fever, anxiety, insomnia? How many non-scientist spouses of scientists can give a clear description of the scientific work in which their partners are engaged? If there is a two-culture gap among the educated, how much wider that gap must be between scientists and those who, for lack of education, are unemployable in an increasingly technological workplace.

The public's high hopes and unrealizable expectations are based partly on ignorance, partly on laziness and self-indulgence; for them, the medical profession has failed to deliver. And yet the profession, ever more obsessed with living up to its part of the social contract, has allowed, indeed encouraged, its medical schools and teaching hospitals to become more and more committed to meeting the social as well as the medical needs of their neighborhoods: their homelessness, poverty, lack of education, addiction to drugs, and crime. With the best of intentions, our medical centers have become burdened with heavy responsibilities that stand well outside their main reason for being—that is, the training of young doctors and the acquisition of new understandings of human biology through research.

ACADEMIC HEALTH CENTERS: JUGGERNAUTS WITHOUT DRIVERS

The first general hospital built in the United States specifically for the care of the sick opened in 1752 in Philadelphia; 13 years later, the first faculty appointment to an American medical school was made by the University of Pennsylvania. The growing together of hospitals, medical schools, and universities proceeded slowly for a century, but the last 100 years have seen a rapid acceleration of merged interests and facilities such that American medicine is now big business.

Today's academic health centers (AHCs) are located mainly in large cities and contain several thousand beds in many different buildings. They service a vast number of out-patients each day; have staffs of thousands; are on duty all day, every day; and have their own power plants, maintenance facilities, security forces, parking lots, shops, multiple feeding facilities, and chapels for various denominations. In fact, they are small cities. Tucked away in each complex is a medical school with as many as 1,000 students and 3,000 full-time faculty members.

The administrators of AHCs must balance the financial books; ensure high standards of professional medical care; see to the training of medical students, residents, and fellows; and answer to a series of local, state, and federal regulators, as well as to their own university authorities. Nothing more is demanded of them than God-like wisdom, judicial balance, financial wizardry, and political genius. But they must be fierce competitors as well. The city and suburban clienteles of patients on whom the AHCs depend to maintain a "full house" are increasingly well served by the many small, non-academic hospitals located in and around the city. Yet certain leaders in U.S. academic medicine think that the horizons of their centers are too limited; they urge still closer working relationships with social scientists, psychologists, lawyers, ethicists, and lay members of the community. They are concerned about the vast numbers of city residents who are under-served, under-insured, under-educated, and under-nourished.

However, a sizable number of thoughtful academics are alarmed by the un-controlled growth of our AHCs, and plead for a re-thinking of the purposes and goals of these organizations. They point to the vast economic problems that burden these centers: Income derived from service to patients, together with endowment income, donations, and governmental support, never seems to keep up with the rising costs of salaries, supplies and equipment, and maintenance. Hitherto, the standard remedies applied by those who subscribe to the modern-day competition model of health care delivery were to increase the in-patient facilities, to overcome the competition of local community hospitals by affiliat-ing with them, and to increase patient-care income by encouraging the utilization of sophisticated technologies that are not yet affordable in smaller hospitals.

Institutional leaders point to the forces that are pulling the AHCs apart: the dominance of the subspecialties of medicine and surgery, and the resultant frag-mentation of authority over teaching and medical service; the loss of collegiality of the professional and paraprofessional staffs, marching to different drummers and less able to speak a common language; the divided loyalties of staff mem-bers, who feel stronger ties to their sources of external funding than to their own deans and department chairmen; and finally, the formation of separate and almost autonomous institutes within a given AHC whose staff members have gained the "privilege" of *not* teaching and *not* rendering service to patients. (Seldin, 1966; Harvey, 1968; Ebert 1986; Rogers, 1986; Chapman, 1987; Ebert and Ginzberg, 1988; Colloton, 1989; Ross and Johns, 1989).

These observers clearly recognize and appreciate the benefits of AHC growth, but their conclusion that the benefits do not outweigh the undesirable side effects of that growth is unmistakable. Deans point with pride to the brilli-ance of their faculty and its ability to bring in grants and contracts, to the growing number of in-patient bed days and out-patient visits, to their ability to provide the costly new technologies that offer the most up-to-date diagnostic and thera-peutic benefits, and to the excitement of participating in an expanding enterprise. But they also recognize that bigness has its price, and they sense that the troubles that academic medicine is facing may have their roots in a loss of mission.

THE FACULTY VIEW

Operating on a different level from their institutional leaders, the faculties of U.S. medical schools are becoming increasingly troubled by the never-slacken-ing demands on their time that reduce their effectiveness as teachers, researchers, or care-givers. These demands are real: Generating income to meet departmental needs has first call on their time. They accomplish this by providing service to private patients that is increasingly procedure-oriented (cardiac catheterization, colonoscopy, computed tomography scans, and so on, because these procedures bring the most money into departmental coffers). But they also must serve on committees that evaluate ethics, guard the rights of experimental animals, police the standards of performance of their colleagues, screen applicants for admission to their medical school, and attend to the forms and reports of outside regulators. What suffers most in this time squeeze is proficiency in teaching. There is too little time for reading or for lively rounds with residents, and as a result, medical teaching has become less stimulating, less exploratory, less inquiring, and more pedestrian (Macy Foundation, 1989).

Increasingly, doctors are saying that the practice of medicine was once enjoyable—but is no longer. *Enjoyment* is a poor word to describe the satisfactions that physician gain from seeing patients: helping people is the motive that has drawn young men and women into medicine. But the boredom of rote learning, uninspired teaching, and hours of being lectured at is likely to convert the idealistic matriculant into a somewhat cynical pragmatist by the time of graduation. Our educational factories are turning out standardized, assembly-line products— men and women who are extremely well informed but not necessarily curious, imaginative, literate, or articulate. In past decades, medical school applicants looked forward to careers in which they would have the independence of being their own bosses; but solo practices are rapidly disappearing, and graduates are increasingly taking salaried positions in group practices as cogs in a larger machine.

In some research-intensive medical schools, faculty members are offered careers in one of three tracks (Kelley, 1988). Traveling in the fast lane is the medical scientist who has won outside grant support and who enjoys "protected time" in which to pursue his research. On a very different track is the skilled clinician who devotes most of his time to seeing patients. The third track is traveled by the faculty member who does both: His research tends to be less demanding of time and skill, and less often is funded by the process of peer review; in addition, he bears the heaviest teaching load with students and residents. In institutions where peer esteem is the coin of the realm, this three-tier system can give rise to jealousies and pecking orders unless great care is taken to reward each tier appropriately. But most research-intensive schools employ only one yardstick for measuring the contributions of the entire staff: the number of articles reporting research results. Clearly, this is an inappropriate yardstick when applied to the teachers and clinicians who are major players in the training of students and residents. The highly trained subspecialist practitioner is rewarded by earning a large income, and the researcher with protected time is rewarded with promotions and tenure. But teachers and skilled clinicians are far less likely to get tenure, and in a research-intensive environment they are less graciously rewarded with a high degree of peer esteem.

Young faculty members who aim at a research career have worries of a different sort. First and foremost, they must acquire training in research methods beyond their clinical training. Their four medical school years are typically choked with course-work that has replaced the laboratory experiences of previous years. Thus, only the students who have had heavy exposure to science in college and the few who have found time during their medical school years to work as apprentices in one of the pre-clinical department laboratories are prepared to go into research after finishing their residencies. There are ways to remedy this lack of training, but, as we shall see, this demands considerable motivation and further years of education. Then, once this second layer of training has been acquired, the young researcher faces long odds in applying for the grant funds needed to support his research; and, if successful, he must compete for funds again every 3–5 years in order to continue that research. The perception of instability and insecurity in this career choice has driven many able young medical graduates away from research and into practice (Movsesian, 1990).

SUMMARY AND CONCLUSIONS

American medicine is in serious trouble today despite the stunning technical advances that have made medical care increasingly effective in the last 40 years. The practice of medicine has been hedged in by bureaucratic regulations at the expense of the loss of professional dependence and personal autonomy; medical education has become rigid, stultified, and depersonalized; medical research has become so expensive that careers in research are no longer attracting bright young doctors; and the provision of medical services to patients has taken on the commercial taint of big business. The public has developed unrealizable expectations for the benefits of quickly available medical treatment and is becoming increasingly litigious when disappointed. Thus, despite the best of intentions, the Social Contract between medicine and the public is becoming increasingly stressed by the burgeoning size and complexity of our AHCs and the rise in the costs of medical care.

The erosion in professionals' confidence in American medicine now runs in parallel with many other social, economic, and political crises; indeed, we seem to be living in a decade of disillusionment, disorganization, and dismay. The problems facing clinical research are only one piece of that larger puzzle, and unless we appreciate the dimensions of American medicine today, we cannot hope to think clearly about the future of clinical research.

2

The Changing Shape of American Medicine

Ten years after the end of World War II, leaders in American medicine concluded that a serious shortage of physicians was imminent. Not only was the general population growing rapidly, but there was an increasing demand for physicians due to recent advances in medical knowledge and skills, and to the development of new physician-intensive technologies. In 1957 the Secretary of the Department of Health, Education and Welfare, Marion B. Folsom, called up a committee of 10 eminent physicians and scientists, chaired by the Dean of the Yale Medical School, Dr. Stanhope Bayne-Jones, to study the role played by the federal government in the nation's health through the U.S. Public Health Service. The committee was asked to project the future need for physicians in light of public requirements and expectations. The Bayne-Jones Report (DHEW Secretary's Consultants 1958) made it clear that there was a pressing need for more doctors and for more medical schools in which to train them. Figures 2–1 and 2–2 show how the number of physicians began to grow in relation to the size of the population, from the plateau of 1950–70 to the unexpectedly large increase in the number of doctors since then. The most recent report of the American Medical Association (AMA) indicates that the number of doctors is still increasing more rapidly than the total population: the annual growth rates are 3.1 and 1.03%, respectively. U.S. doctors now number about 230 per 100,000 population; for comparison, Japan has 157 doctors per 100,000 population; the United Kingdom, 164; West Germany, 256; Sweden, 264; Spain, 313; France, 319; Belgium, 302; and Italy, 424. Thus, the United States is among the nations with the highest number of physicians per unit of population, but it is by no means the highest (if we can credit these 1988 World Health Organization (WHO) figures).

The U.S. Census Bureau does its best to count the number of people living in the 50 states; these tallies are made extremely difficult owing to unknown numbers of illegal aliens, the homeless, and other residents who resist being counted. The number of U.S. physicians, on the other hand, is known with great precision due to the fastidious work of the AMA, which has an elaborate system of naming and tracking all U.S. doctors, whether active or retired. The primary record is a self-administered questionnaire mailed to all physicians every 4 years.

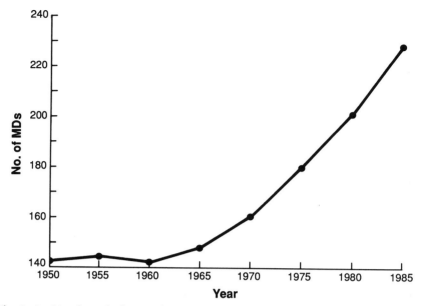

Fig. 2–1   Number of *all* U.S. physicians per 100,000 population. (*AMA Physician Characteristics and Distribution in the United States,* 1986, Table A–7)

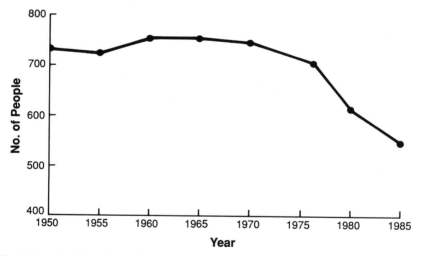

Fig. 2–2   Number of people per *active* physician in the United States. (*AMA Physician Characteristics and Distribution in the United States,* 1986, Table A–7)

The information provided on this questionnaire is confirmed by the data obtained on individuals through their various affiliations: medical societies, specialty boards, hospitals, and so on. The questionnaire, called the Record of Physicians' Professional Activities, requests the usual demographic data but, in addition, asks whether the respondent's practice is office- or hospital-based. It also requires each doctor to estimate the number of hours spent in five different activities (described in detail below) and to state whether he concentrates his practice in one or more special disciplines or specialties. This ongoing survey process is updated, corrected, and added to almost daily. Any inaccuracies are due to wrong or missing addresses and to incomplete replies. The managers of this elaborate informational network think that the degree of unreliability now hovers between 3 and 4%.

The resultant AMA Physician Masterfile is capable of breaking out analyses of many kinds: total numbers of MDs, inactive MDs (for various reasons of age, health, or inclination); number of MDs who concentrate their practices in any of some 35 tabulated specialties and subspecialties; number of MDs who are board certified by one or more of the twenty-three American Specialty Boards; as well as ethnic, racial, and gender data, and many other tabulations filling an annual publication totaling more than 200 pages. And because the AMA has been performing these counts for many years, changes over time can be plotted in order to evaluate how the activities of U.S. physicians are evolving in response to changes in training, employment opportunities, governmental regulations, technical advances, or other factors.

The latest figures in the AMA Physician Masterfile (1989) show a grand total of about 600,000 MDs (Table 2–1) of whom 89% are active and validly classifiable in terms of their primary activity. "Primary activity" is defined as one of the five activities in which the respondent spends the most professional time (a plurality tabulation):

1. Patient care: hours spent in seeing patients and/or rendering patient services, whether office-based or hospital-based (includes interns, residents, clinical trainees, and clinical fellows).
2. Medical teaching: hours spent teaching or preparing to teach in medical schools, hospitals, nursing schools, or other institutions of higher learning.
3. Medical research: hours spent in activities (funded or unfunded) performed to develop new medical knowledge that is potentially publishable (includes physicians in research fellowship programs).
4. Administration: hours spent as a salaried staff member or executive in a hospital, health facility, health agency, clinic, group, or any other health-oriented organization.
5. Other: hours spent in medical activities not listed above and not involving direct care of patients (such as employment by insurance carriers, corporations, pharmaceutical companies, voluntary organizations, medical

Table 2–1   Federal and Non-Federal Physicians in the U.S. (1989)

Total Number

Graduates of U.S. medical schools	461,919	
Graduates of Canadian medical schools	8,209	
Graduates of other foreign medical schools	129,340	
Graduates of presently inactive medical schools	1,321	
		600,789

Total Number of Active Physicians

Exclusive of 64,034 MDs (the sum of inactive plus address unknown plus non-classifiable)	536,755

Primary Activity of Active Physicians

		% of Total Active
Patient care	493,159	91.9
Medical teaching	8,196	1.5
Medical research	16,941	3.2
Administration	14,767	2.8
Other	3,692	0.7
Total	536,755	

Source: AMA Physician Masterfile, Department of Physician Data Services, January 1, 1989.

societies, or associations; or work in health-related journalism, law, or sales).

Table 2–1 presents the number of U.S. physicians and their medical school origins in 1989: 600,789 total, 77% of whom were trained in U.S. medical schools. Physicians validly classified as active numbered 536,755, or 89% of the total number on record; 91.9% of these were engaged primarily in patient care. Of interest is the fact that twice as many physicians claim to spend the majority of their time in medical research compared to medical teaching. (We will return later to other estimates of the number of doctors engaged in research.)

Table 2–2 shows that from 1969 to 1987, the total number of active MDs rose from 305,047 to 537,555—a 76% increase—but the numbers in teaching, administration, and research changed very little. The data in the far right column, which are a measure of the degree of reliability of the Masterfile information, show a ninefold variation (from 1.1 to 10.0% unclassified and unknown address) that correlates inversely with the small shifts in the proportion of doctors in patient care: that percentage hovered around 88–90% in the years when the error data were smallest.

The AMA Physician Masterfile for 1989 also documents that 20,359 physicians, or 4% of all active physicians, had positions in the federal government (the military services, Veterans Administration, U.S. Public Health Service, Peace Corps), and that 344,671 physicians of all U.S. physicians (57%) were board certified by one or more of the 23 specialty boards.

To recapitulate, then, there are some 600,000 active MDs in the United

Table 2–2 Primary Activity of Physicians in the United States (1969–87)[a]

Fiscal Year	Total Number of Active Physicians[b]	Patient Care		Medical Teaching		Administration		Medical Research		Other		Unclassified and Unknown Address	
		N	%	N	%	N	%	N	%	N	%	N	%
1969	305,047	270,737	88.8	5,149	1.7	12,107	4.0	12,375	4.1	2,598	0.9	5,865	1.9
1970	314,407	278,535	88.6	5,588	1.8	12,158	3.9	11,929	3.8	2,635	0.8	3,562	1.1
1971	325,435		88.3		1.8		3.7		3.3		0.8		2.1
1972	336,424		86.9		1.7		3.3		2.8		0.8		4.6
1973	343,755		85.9		1.8		3.5		2.4		0.8		5.6
1974	358,134		84.1		1.7		3.3		2.2		0.7		7.8
1975	372,293	311,937	83.8	6,445	1.7	11,161	3.0	7,944	2.1	2,793	0.8	32,013	8.6
1976	387,329		82.2		1.7		3.0		2.2		0.7		10.0
1977	392,913		84.6		1.7		3.0		2.5		0.7		7.5
1978	410,655		83.6		1.7		2.9		2.8		0.7		8.5
1979	426,226		83.7		1.8		2.8		3.4		0.7		7.6
1980	441,935	376,512	85.2	7,942	1.6	12,209	2.8	15,377	3.5	2,876	0.7	27,019	6.1
1981	450,112		86.5		1.6		2.9		4.0		0.7		4.3
1982	466,268		87.6		1.6		2.9		3.6		0.7		3.6
1983	482,635		87.7		1.6		2.9		3.8		0.7		3.3
1984	500,553		87.3		1.6		2.8		4.6		0.7		3.1
1985	514,070	448,820	87.3	7,832	1.5	13,810	2.7	23,268	4.5	3,410	0.7	16,930	3.3
1986	522,325	462,126	88.5	7,721	1.5	14,399	2.8	17,847	3.4	3,657	0.7	16,575	3.2
1987	537,555	478,511	89.0	8,114	1.5	14,536	2.7	16,586	3.1	3,581	0.7	16,227	3.1

[a]From AMA *Physician Characteristics*, with data after 1968 when the classification system was most recently revised.
[b]Excludes inactive doctors and those living temporarily abroad, but includes "Unclassified and Unknown Address."

States, nearly 92% of whom work primarily in patient care; this proportion has not changed over the last 20 years, even though the total number of physicians has risen by 75%. Those in medical administration and medical research number about 14,500 and 16,500, respectively—about 6% of the total—and more than half of all U.S. physicians are board-certified specialists. Only about 8,000 MDs claim that medical teaching is their primary activity; this surprisingly low number leads us to consider our 127 U.S. medical schools.

U.S. MEDICAL SCHOOLS: THEIR STUDENTS AND FACULTIES

The Flexner Report (1910) dealt in detail with the 155 medical schools then extant in the United States and Canada, all of which Flexner visited personally and surveyed in terms of their faculties, students, physical facilities, tuition charges, and curriculum. His detailed description of the for-profit status and low educational standards of many of the schools led to closures, and to reforms among those that remained in action. By 1925 there were some 80 U.S. schools (of which more than 15 were not fully accredited). In 1958, when the Bayne-Jones Report called for the formation of at least 10 new schools, there were 77 schools (only 2 on probation), growing to 95 fully accredited schools in 1969 and to 127 in 1982—a total that still stands. The rapid growth in the number of medical schools after 1969 was due to federal funding of construction costs and of sizable allowances based on the number of students admitted (capitation allowances). Today 74 of the 127 schools are public and 53 are private; the large growth in state schools has been made possible by both federal and local funds.

U.S. medical schools vary enormously in many ways. In 1987–88, the number of medical students per 4-year school varied from 92 to 1,303, and the number of master's and doctoral degree candidates training in the pre-clinical departments of those schools varied from 0 to 465. Faculties (total full-time) ranged in size from 40 to 3,006; annual revenues from $4.4 million to $574 million; and annual operating costs from $3.6 million to $493 million. [These data appear in the *Institutional Profile System* of the Association of American Medical Colleges (AAMC).]

Applicants to U.S. Medical Schools

Recent declines in the number of applicants to U.S. medical schools have been the source of great concern to medical educators, but it is useful to view this decline historically. Figure 2–3 shows the rapid increase in the number of students enrolled per year after 1969, leveling off after 1980. But it also shows large variations in the number of applicants, with a sudden burst after World War II (induced in part by the Servicemen's Readjustment Act of 1944, commonly known as the GI Bill of Rights) and a second larger increase starting in the late 1960s that reflected the federal government's perception of an impending shortage of doctors and the resultant formation of new schools with larger class en-

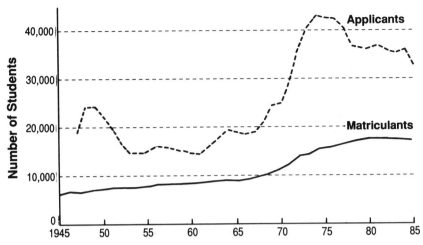

Fig. 2–3 Medical school applicants and matriculants, 1945–85. (*AAMC Report on American Medical Education: Institutions, Characteristics and Programs*, 1986, Fig. 8)

rollments. Table 2–3 gives the numerical data on medical school enrollments and numbers of graduates in 5-year periods from 1925 to 1973, and annually from 1973 to 1988, the period of current concern. From 1925 to 1973 the ratio of applicants to acceptances has ranged from a low of 1.65 in 1925–28 to a high of 2.96 in 1949–53. From 1973 to the present, the ratio fell slowly but steadily, from 2.83 to its lowest, of 1.56, in 1988.

Before leaving Table 2–3, note that the numbers of graduates from U.S. medical schools increased from 4,262 in 1925–28 to its maximum of 16,343 in 1983, a fourfold increase in output from schools that increased in number only from 80 to 127. Over that 63-year period, mean class size increased from 53 to 129, with the largest individual graduating class today totaling 284. The effect of these changes, in terms of quality of education, will be considered later.

So much for quantity: what about the quality of the applicants to U.S. medical schools? A number of educators have perceived a decline in the quality of applicants in recent years, based partly on their personal contacts with students (an assessment that may be biased by generational differences in lifestyle) and partly on small declines in the standardized test scores that applicants submit to admissions committees. Figs. 2–4 and 2–5 plot the changes between 1981 and 1988 in the grade point averages (GPAs) achieved by applicants and matriculants to medical schools during their undergraduate college years. The overall scores for *all* courses and, separately, those for *science* courses show the same trends, with higher scores for matriculants in 1981 than in 1988. However, these differences in *mean* GPAs seem trivial when viewed alongside the numerical data in Table 2–4. In this table, the standard deviations (SDs) of the means are sufficiently large that the differences between the means could easily have been due to chance. Again, the scores of the matriculants were higher than those of the

the applicants (though not significantly higher), which presumably reflects the admissions committees' selection process.

Applicants to medical schools are subjected to standardized aptitude tests called Medical College Admission Tests (MCATs), the scores of which are used by admissions committees in screening their applicant pools, along with other indicators of suitability for admittance to medical schools, such as letters of reference, participation in extracurricular activities, and personal interviews. Again, as Table 2–4 shows, there appear to be no significant differences in the 1981 and 1988 MCAT scores of applicants and matriculants, given the wide spread of the SDs in each of the six test categories.

Thus, for both GPAs and MCATs, the trends may seem more alarming than real. However, a possibly more valid concern stems from the marked change since 1975 in the selections by college undergraduates of their major fields of concentration. Table 2–5 (last column to the right) shows large increases in the number of baccalaureate degrees awarded in the fields of computer and administration services, engineering, and business management, but striking decreases in the number of these degrees awarded in the life sciences (along with declines in literature, social sciences, and education). This fall-off in the number of college students majoring in the life sciences foretells a shrinkage in the number of prospective medical school applicants a few years later; this is indeed an indicator that bears close watching.

Faculties of U.S. Medical Schools

Just as the annual growth rate of the U.S. physician population has exceeded that of the population at large, the growth in the number of full-time faculty in U.S. medical schools has outstripped that of the student body. Since 1969, when the rate of formation of new medical schools escalated from 101 to 127, along with larger annual enrollments, the annual growth rate of full-time faculty members has been more than double that of first-year medical school matriculants (5.9 vs. 2.7%); the largest part of this faculty increase has taken place in the clinical departments (83% of the entire increase). In 1969 the ratio of full-time faculty to first-year matriculants was 2.37; in 1989 it was 4.19. And although the number of medical schools and the number of medical students graduating annually has shown little or no change over the last 10 years, the full-time faculty has continued to increase from 46,662 to 70,308 (a 4.2% annual growth rate); 91% of that increase took place in the clinical departments. (The implications of this increase will become more apparent when we discuss the growing need for income-generation in the clinical departments.)

Since World War II, the major responsibility for teaching medical students, residents, and clinical fellows has been delegated to full-time faculty members as the teaching role of part-time faculty has been intentionally scaled down. However, the number of doctors who serve our medical schools as part-time salaried faculty members and unpaid volunteer faculty members should not be overlooked. The 1989 AMA report on undergraduate medical education (Jonas

Table 2-5 BA Degrees Conferred by Institutions of Higher Education in Selected Disciplines (1975–76 to 1984–85)

Discipline	1975–76		1978–79		1981–82		1984–85		Percent Change, 1976–85
	Number	Percent	Number	Percent	Number	Percent	Number	Percent	
Total, all degrees	925,426	100	921,390	100	952,998	100	979,477	100	5.8
Total, selected degrees	668,528	72.1	655,218	71.1	682,336	71.6	703,854	71.9	5.3
Computer and Admin. Services	5,652	0.6	8,719	0.9	20,267	2.1	36,867	3.8	552.3
Engineering	38,388	4.1	53,021	5.8	67,021	7.0	77,154	7.9	100.1
Business management	142,379	15.4	171,764	18.6	214,001	22.5	233,351	23.8	63.9
Health sciences[a]	53,813	5.8	61,819	6.7	63,385	6.7	64,513	6.6	19.9
Psychology	49,908	5.4	42,461	4.6	41,031	4.3	39,811	4.1	−20.2
English language and literature	43,019	4.6	34,557	3.8	34,334	3.6	34,091	3.5	−20.8
Social sciences	126,287	13.6	107,922	11.7	99,545	10.4	91,461	9.3	−27.6
Life sciences[b]	54,275	5.9	48,846	5.3	41,639	4.4	38,445	3.9	−29.2
Education	154,807	16.7	126,109	13.7	101,113	10.6	88,161	9.0	−43.1

[a]Mainly nursing, health administration, and health technologies.

[b]Mainly pre-medical and pre-dental students.

Source: DHHS Report to the President and Congress: Sixth report on the status of health personnel in the United States, June 1988, Table 2-6, derived from 1987 and earlier editions of the U.S. Department of Education's *Digest of Education Statistics*.

Table 2–3 Medical School Applicants, Enrollment, and Graduates (1925–88)

Years	Number of Schools	Applicants	Accepted Applicants	Applicants/ Acceptance Ratio	Graduates
1925–28	80	10,769	6,458	1.65	4,262
1929–33	76	12,785	7,062	1.77	4,715
1934–38	77	12,409	6,954	1.76	5,178
1939–43	77	12,354	6,484	1.84	5,169
1949–53*	79	21,528	7,364	2.96	5,906
1954–58	83	15,172	8,034	1.88	6,868
1959–63	91	14,947	8,616	1.76	7,074
1964–68	92	18,503	9,189	2.00	7,607
1969–73	108	27,175	11,646	2.32	9,071
1974	114	42,624	15,066	2.83	12,716
1975	114	42,303	15,365	2.70	13,634
1976	116	42,155	15,774	2.70	13,614
1977	122	40,569	15,977	2.50	14,391
1978	125	36,636	16,527	2.20	14,966
1979	126	36,141	16,886	2.10	15,135
1980	126	36,100	17,146	2.10	15,673
1981	126	36,727	17,286	2.10	15,985
1982	127	35,730	17,294	2.10	15,802
1983	127	35,200	17,209	2.00	16,343
1984	127	35,944	17,194	2.10	16,318
1985	127	32,893	17,228	1.90	16,117
1986	127	31,323	17,092	1.80	15,830
1987	127	28,123	17,027	1.70	15,919
1988	127	26,721	17,108	1.56	16,341

*Data incomplete for the years 1944–49.

Sources: Schofield (1984), Table 2; AAMC (personal communication, Donna J. Williams, Section for Operational Studies).

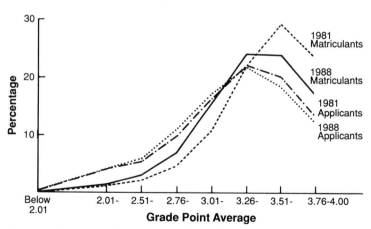

Fig. 2–4 Overall grade point averages of applicants and matriculants, 1981 and 1988. (*AAMC Report on Medical School Applicants and Matriculants: Trends, 1981–88*)

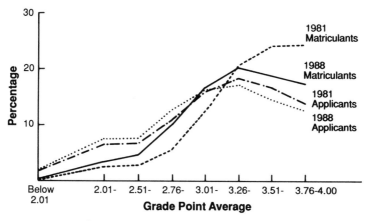

Fig. 2–5 Science grade point averages of applicants and matriculants, 1981 and 1988. (*AAMC Report on Medical School Applicants and Matriculants: Trends, 1981–88*)

Table 2–4 GPAs and MCAT Scores of Applicants and Matriculants to U.S. Medical Schools (1981 and 1988)

	1981		1988	
	Applicants	Matriculants	Applicants	Matriculants
GPAs[a]				
Science	3.24	3.46	3.19	3.34
	± 0.50	± 0.40	± 0.51	± 0.43
Overall	3.31	3.50	3.29	3.42
	± 0.42	± 0.34	± 0.42	± 0.36
MCAT Scores[b]				
Biology	8.65	9.66	8.83	9.62
	± 2.36	± 1.91	± 2.28	± 1.85
Chemistry	8.57	9.69	8.54	9.37
	± 2.37	± 2.04	± 2.40	± 2.10
Physics	8.55	9.65	8.56	9.39
	± 2.48	± 2.24	± 2.50	± 2.22
Science problems	8.50	9.61	8.50	9.35
	± 2.39	± 2.08	± 2.40	± 2.08
Reading skills	8.22	8.94	8.03	8.68
	± 2.30	± 1.87	± 2.36	± 1.92
Quantitative skills	8.10	9.02	8.03	8.72
	± 2.42	± 2.16	± 2.40	± 2.15

[a]Scored from 0 to 4.0, as averages ± one standard deviation.

[b]Scored from 1 to 15, as averages ± one standard deviation.

Source: *AAMC Report on Medical School Applicants: Trends*, 1981–88, pp. 22–25 and 42–47.

et al., 1989) noted that 137,200 faculty members served in these capacities, along with 9,837 paid part-timers and 127,363 volunteers. This brought the total number of faculty members (paid and unpaid) in our 127 medical schools to 207,508 in 1988. Data on part-time and volunteer faculty are available only since 1972. In the last 17 years, there has been an approximate doubling in the number of full-time faculty, while the number of paid part-time faculty has remained quite constant at 8,000–10,000. Thus, the proportion of paid part-timers today is about one-eighth of the total full-time faculty, while in 1972 it was about one-third. [The history of the development of the full-time faculty system, beginning in the United States in the first years of this century at Johns Hopkins, and the implications of this radical policy change for teaching and research, have been described in detail by Fye (1991).]

Looking now at the division of total full-time faculty between the pre-clinical and clinical faculties and the changes in those proportions since 1961, Table 2–6 presents the data for 1961 to 1988; Fig. 2–6 shows these trends graphically. It is seen that most of the growth rate of faculty members in U.S. medical schools has been due to steadily increasing numbers in the clinical departments, with an annual growth of 7.6% since 1961 compared to 4.8% in the pre-clinical departments. These changes should be considered in light of the diminishing influence of part-time faculty in medical school activities in recent years. Fifty years ago, much of the teaching and service to patients was performed by part-time faculty; this is no longer the case.

The sources of these data must be described in order to judge their quality. Data on the number of full-time faculty members of the 127 U.S. medical schools are gathered by two agencies, the AAMC and the AMA. AAMC questionnaires are addressed to individual faculty members and kept updated by administrative representatives of the AAMC at each school; AMA data are collected through reports filed annually by each dean's office with the AMA's Liaison Committee on Medical Education (LCME). For each system, an annual report is published: the AAMC's *Faculty Roster System: Numbers Book* and the AMA's annual report on undergraduate medical education, published in *JAMA*. The Faculty Roster System is considered to be about 85% complete and up-to-date; the LCME data are considered to be more than 95% complete. The comparability of these two data sources can be seen in Table 2–7 for the academic year 1987–88. The agreement between the AAMC and AMA data is quite good, considering the different mechanisms applied in gathering them and the 85% reliability estimate placed by the AAMC on its Faculty Roster System process.

Table 2–7 also shows that in 1987–88 some 40,000 individuals with MD degrees were employed full-time in U.S. medical schools. Further, these 127 schools employed about 17,000 PhDs and some 3,500 individuals with other degrees. Thus, the pre-clinical departments made up about 20% of the faculty and clinical departments 78%. In the tables and figures below, we will see how these numbers and proportions have changed over the last 20 years.

Table 2–8 shows that since 1970 (when such data first became available), the proportion of PhDs in the full-time faculties of U.S. medical schools has

Table 2–6 Full-Time Faculty in All U.S. Medical Schools, 1961–1988

Fiscal Year	Number of Schools	Faculty Numbers			% in Clinical Depts.
		Total	Pre-Clinical Depts.	Clinical Depts.	
1961	86	11,224	4,023	7,201	64.2
1962	86	12,040	4,342	7,698	63.9
1963	87	13,602	4,693	8,909	66.0
1964	88	15,015	5,541	9,474	63.1
1965	89	15,882	5,233	10,649	67.1
1966	89	17,118	5,671	11,447	66.9
1967	92	19,297	5,877	13,420	69.5
1968	99	22,293	6,639	15,654	70.2
1969	101	23,034	7,048	15,986	69.4
1970	103	24,093	7,287	16,806	69.8
1971	108	27,539	8,283	19,256	69.9
1972	112	30,170	8,714	21,456	71.1
1973	114	33,265	9,381	23,884	71.8
1974	114	34,878	9,928	24,950	71.5
1975	114	37,010	10,164	26,846	72.5
1976	116	39,346	10,743	28,603	72.7
1977	122	41,650	11,301	30,349	72.9
1978	125	44,358	11,736	32,622	73.5
1979	126	46,662	12,605	34,057	73.0
1980	126	49,446	12,831	36,665	74.2
1981	126	50,532	12,816	37,716	74.6
1982	127	53,371	13,223	40,148	75.2
1983	127	55,525	13,587	41,938	75.5
1984	127	57,003	13,560	43,443	76.2
1985	127	58,774	13,767	45,007	76.6
1986	127	61,397	14,204	47,193	76.9
1987	127	63,313	14,479	48,834	77.1
1988	127	66,798	14,580	52,218	78.2
1989	127	70,308	14,832	55,476	78.9
Annual growth rate (1961–89)	1.4%	6.7%	4.8%	7.6%	

Sources: IOM-NAS *Committee Report on Personnel Needs and Training for Biomedical and Behavioral Research* (1985), Appendix Table A2. Updated for 1984–89 by Dr. Charles R. Sherman, Office of the Director, NIH, based on data supplied by the AMA.

remained unchanged at about 29%. This is of interest in view of the increasing number of research grants awarded to PhDs over those years (for details, see Chapter 7).

MDs are increasingly clustered in the clinical departments. Table 2–9 shows that in 1970 over 85% of all MDs were so assigned; in 1988, 93%. However, the converse is *not* the case. PhDs are no longer employed so dominantly in the *pre*-clinical departments. In 1988, about 45% of the PhD faculty members were

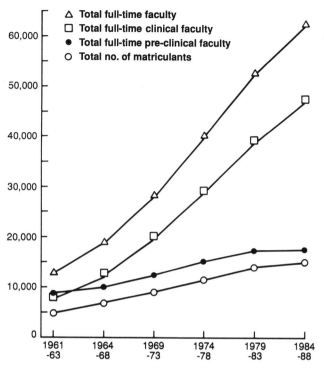

Fig. 2–6 Number of matriculants and full-time faculty in U.S. medical schools, 1961–88. (AAMC, Donna J. Williams, Section for Operational Studies, personal communication)

working exclusively in clinical departments, an increase from about 36% in 1970. The significance of this change will become clear in later pages.

Herman and Singer (1986) reported that the number of PhDs employed in clinical departments in U.S. medical schools was increasing more rapidly than the number of MD's. On the basis of data generated by them from the AAMC Faculty Roster System, they reported that over the period 1972–82, the number of PhDs in clinical departments had increased at a rate of 6.5% per year, compared to 5.0% for MDs. However, in their calculations, they chose to lump all pathologists (MDs and PhDs) into the clinical department category, even though many medical schools count their pathologists as members of the pre-clinical faculty. Where to assign pathologists (clinical or pre-clinical) is an arbitrary decision, for certain of their activities are performed in both disciplines. For instance, the first exposure to pathology is usually considered part of a medical student's pre-clinical education, whereas the performance of autopsies and the examination of surgical biopsy specimens are closely related to the clinical affairs of the hospitals in which they are carried out.

There appears to be no evidence to dispute the conclusion that PhDs are

Table 2–7 Distribution of Full-Time Faculty in U.S. Medical Schools and Affiliated Hospitals in the Academic Year 1987–88

	AAMC[a]	AMA[b]
Total number of faculty positions (filled)	60,534	66,798
MDs	36,881	
MD-PhDs	3,319	
PhDs	16,777	
Other degrees	3,577	
Positions (filled) in pre-clinical departments	11,960	14,580
MDs	2,143	
MD-PhDs	694	
PhDs	8,703	
Other degrees	420	
Positions (filled) in clinical departments	46,969	52,218
MDs	34,449	
MD-PhDs	2,589	
PhDs	7,327	
Other degrees	2,604	
Positions (filled) in other assignments	1,605	—
Grand Totals	60,534	66,798

Sources:
[a]*AAMC Faculty Roster System: Numbers Book* (1988).
[b]Jonas and Etzel (1988).

Table 2–8 Lack of Change in Proportions of MDs and PhDs in Full-Time Faculties of U.S. Medical Schools at 3-Year Intervals (1970–88)[a]

	MDs[b]		PhDs	
	Number	%	Number	%
1970	18,199	71.8	7,154	28.2
1973	22,021	70.6	9,153	29.4
1976	26,912	70.8	11,100	29.2
1979	31,213	71.0	12,757	29.0
1982	35,168	71.2	14,236	28.8
1985	37,816	71.5	15,038	28.5
1988	40,333	71.9	15,786	28.1

[a]Exclusive of degree holders other than MDs, MD-PhDs, and PhDs. Other degree holders varied from 12.1% of total full-time faculty in 1970 to 6.6% in 1988.
[b]Includes MD-PhDs.
Source: Personal communication, Joan Bailey, Office of the Director, NIH, July 1989.

Table 2–9   Faculty affiliations of MDs and PhDs in U.S. Medical Schools, in 1970 and 1988[a]

	MDs[b]			PhDs		
		Percentages in:			Percentages in:	
	Total No.	Pre-Clinical Depts.	Clinical Depts.	Total No.	Pre-Clinical Depts.	Clinical Depts.
1970	18,199	14.6	85.4	7,154	64.2	35.8
1988	40,333	7.1	92.9	15,786	54.9	45.1

[a]Exclusive of degree holders other than MDs, MD-PhDs, and PhDs.
[b]Includes MD-PhDs.
Source: Personal communication, Joan Bailey, Office of the Director, NIH, July 1989.

increasingly being employed in clinical departments, even when the AAMC Faculty Roster System data are accepted as given them by offices of their school members, and are not manipulated, as Herman and Singer did. What remains uncertain is the magnitude of the increase.

What may be of greater interest, however, are the wide disparities among the several clinical departments in their hiring patterns of MDs and PhDs. Data collected by Sherman (1989) (Office of the Director, National Institutes of Health, NIH) and discussed in more detail in Chapter 5 refer to the numbers of the various degree holders in the many separate pre-clinical and clinical departments in FY 1987. This compilation was made possible by linking the AAMC Faculty Roster data with the NIH IMPAC database, thus overcoming the inability of the former to identify the research activity of its individual faculty members and the inability of the latter to identify the departmental affiliation of NIH grant awardees. Setting aside the question of assigning pathology faculty members to pre-clinical or clinical departments, or both, Sherman's data show that the proportions of PhDs employed in *other* clinical departments varied from 5.9% in anesthesiology to 33.0% in psychiatry and 41.3% in public health, with a mean of 18.4% ($\pm$ 10.1). In order of size of the clinical departments, medicine employed 9.4% of its faculty as PhDs, pediatrics and surgery 10.7%, and psychiatry 33.0%, these four departments accounting for 63% of the total clinical faculty in U.S. medical schools. (Of course, these averages conceal large variations in the research, teaching, and service priorities of one school compared to another, and thus in their employment of PhDs.)

These wide variations in the employment of PhDs in clinical departments raise important questions. What are the special skills that these scientists bring to their departments? And is their role in these departments that of a research leader or follower? In psychiatry and public health, PhDs unquestionably bring the expertise of psychology, sociology, economics, law, and ethics to assist their MD colleagues; in medicine and pediatrics, they add the skills of biochemistry, molecular and cell biology, and biostatistics. As to whether they are leaders or followers, I know of no discerning examination of this question. Suffice it to say here that 27% of the PhDs in clinical departments were principal investigators (PIs) on NIH grants in fiscal year 1987, compared to 11% of the MDs. These figures indicate what a mistake it would be to consider PhDs in clinical departments merely as individuals hired to perform laboratory work that the MD's have less and less time for, or simply as supervisors of technicians in those laboratories.

In summary, then, the total growth of full-time faculties has proceeded at the rate of about 7% per year since 1961, with growth in the clinical departments outstripping that in the pre-clinical departments by 2:1. PhDs are increasingly invited to accept appointments in clinical departments, but at widely varying rates among the several clinical departments and from one school to another. Their value to these departments is in no way measured by these changing employment rates.

REVENUES OF U.S. MEDICAL SCHOOLS

Some considerations of the total revenues of U.S. medical schools and their sources is germane to this book for at least two reasons. First, the funding by government (federal, state, and local) has been heavy since the early 1960s, and this carries with it the right of oversight on behalf of the taxpayers. Until 1975, government funds made up more than 50% of total medical school revenues. In later years, however, the rate of growth in governmental contributions slowed greatly in constant dollars as well as in the proportionate share of total revenues. Second, the increases in tuition and fees demanded by all medical schools (public as well as private) have burdened the families of medical students and contributed to the declining number of applicants, yet this source makes up less than 6% of the total revenues of U.S. medical schools.

The overall trends in sources of revenue are illustrated in Fig. 2–7, which shows the dramatic rise in revenues from medical service since 1975 and the relatively small contribution of tuition to total revenues. For the individual matriculant, however, the up-front costs of a 4-year medical education loom very large. According to the AAMC (1990 *AAMC Data Book,* Table E1), the median annual cost of tuition plus fees (the part of a student's expenses that goes to the school) was $17,000 in 1988 for the 53 private schools and $5,575 for public schools' state residents (and $11,700 for out-of-state residents). In constant dollars, the cost of 4 years' medical schooling has risen since 1960 more than 4-fold for students in private schools, 3.5-fold for out-of-state students in public schools, and 2.8-fold for in-state students in public schools. Most students borrow to meet these costs. The 1989 *JAMA* report on undergraduate medical education (Jonas et al., 1989) states that 83.4% of medical students have educational debts. The trends in their indebtedness are shown in Fig. 2–8 up to 1984–85. In current dollars, the 1988 graduates had a mean debt of $38,489 (an 8% increase

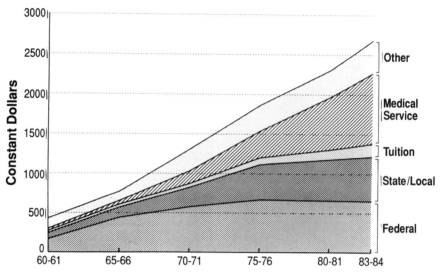

Fig. 2–7 Distribution of sources of revenues for medical schools, 1961–84 (in millions of 1960 dollars). (*AAMC Report on American Medical Education: Institutions, Characteristics and Programs,* 1986, Fig. 4)

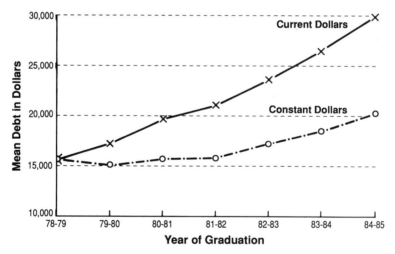

Fig. 2–8 Mean debt of indebted medical school graduates, 1979–85 (in current and 1979 dollars). (*AAMC Report on American Medical Education: Institutions, Characteristics and Programs,* 1986, Fig. 11)

over the 1987 figure). For public school students it was $31,370, and for private school students it was $48,068.

It is revealing to compare the revenue picture of private medical schools with that of private universities that do not have medical schools. This comparison highlights the pivotal role of tuition income for private universities and the equally pivotal role of medical service income for private medical schools. Table 2–10 shows these comparisons. Medical schools derive 44.8% of their revenues from sources unique to their role as producers of health services, while private universities without medical schools depend most heavily on tuition (57%).

Since 1970, the trends on revenue sources of all U.S. medical schools at

Table 2–10 Sources of Revenues of Private U.S. Universities Compared to Those of Private Medical Schools, 1985–86

	Revenue Sources of	
	Private Medical Schools[a]	Private Universities without Medical Schools[b]
	(as percentages of total revenues)	
Tuition and fees	7.6	57.0
Federal sources	25.0	13.1
Grants, contracts, appropriations	17.6	
Indirect cost recovery	7.4	
Private gifts and grants	1.2	13.2
Endowment income	2.3	8.4
State and local govt. sources	5.8	2.2
Appropriations	3.3	
Sponsored programs	2.7	
Indirect cost recovery	0.9	
Revenues unique to U.S. medical schools	44.8	
Research and training programs in affiliated institutions	1.1	
Hospital reimbursements	21.2	
Professional fee income	22.5	
Miscellaneous	13.3	6.2
University funds	1.0	
College service income	0.8	
Nongovt. sponsored programs	8.8	
Other	2.7	
Total	100.0%	100.0%

[a]Revenues of all 53 private U.S. medical schools totaled $4,965 million.

Source: Jolly et al. (1988), Table 9.

[b]Revenues of all 363 private universities without medical schools totaled $6,714 million.

Source: DOE State Higher Education Profiles (1988), Table 5, p. 23.

Table 2–11   Trends in U.S. Medical School Revenues (in millions of 1987 dollars)[a]

	1970–71		1980–81		1987–88	
	Amt.	%	Amt.	%	Amt.	%
Federal research	1,391	25.6	2,265	22.5	2,873	20.4
Other federal	1,023	18.8	620	6.2	488	3.5
State and local govts.	1,026	18.9	2,274	22.6	2,477	17.6
Tuition & fees	200	3.7	542	5.4	722	5.1
Professional service	664	12.2	2,898	28.8	5,428	38.5
Other income	1,137	20.9	1,465	14.6	2,118	15.0
Total	5,442	100.0	10,064	100.0	14,106	100.0

[a]All schools, public and private.
Source: Taksel et al. (1989), Table 4.

three time points are shown in Table 2–11 in 1987 dollars. Over that 17-year period, total revenues in constant dollars increased nearly threefold. Total federal dollars increased 39%, but their share of total revenues decreased from 44 to 24%, while professional service income rose from 12 to 39%.

The impact of an increasing need for professional service income on education and research in U.S. medical schools over the last 20 years will be taken up in greater detail later. Suffice it to say here that professional service income is the engine driving our medical schools today. The rapidly growing need for this income has affected the hiring of medical school faculties, as well as the allotment of professional time for education and research by clinical faculties. Of the three major functions of the medical schools, it is obvious that service pays its way and more; research pays a very large part of its costs through grants and indirect cost disbursements. But education? That is an untold story: The costs of undergraduate medical education per se have never been disentangled from those for research, service, and administration.

AHCs AND GRADUATE MEDICAL EDUCATION

The medical education of U.S.-trained physicians does not end with graduation from medical school, nor even after the single year of hospital experience that all states require for licensure to practice. Another 3 or 4 years of postgraduate hospital training must be undertaken by all who aspire to become board-certified in medicine or pediatrics (and 1 or 2 more years for subspecialty training) and, for surgery, 6 or more postgraduate years. Thus, the professional education of doctors occurs in three stages—college, medical school, and hospital residency—each independently designed, operated, and sited. This process is familiarly known as the "4-4-4 system." It has evolved over time to satisfy the standards of excellence demanded by the specialty boards and by the governing boards of the nearly 6,000 U.S. hospitals to which doctors must apply for admission privileges. Because of the lack of integration among the three elements of the 4-4-4 system, and because of the increasing concern over the length of time taken to bring a young person through the medical education process and out into the real world, the 4-4-4 system has come under severe criticism by educators who think that the entire process can not only be shortened but also vastly improved in quality (Ebert and Ginzberg, 1988). Their arguments focus mainly on the educational deficiencies of this tripartite system, and on the undesirable results of the growing imbalance among the three missions of our medical schools and teaching hospitals (education, service to patients, and research).

All hospitals in the United States must be accredited by the medical, hospital, and nursing associations in order to keep their doors open to the public. The accreditation review is performed by a visiting team every 3 years, which looks for violations and for satisfactory correction of previously noted problems. According to the AAMC, there were 5,622 accredited hospitals in the United States in 1989, 46% of which had fewer than 100 beds and 5% of which had more than 500 beds (chronic care and federal hospitals are not included in this tally). Of these 5,622 hospitals, 1,285 are called "teaching hospitals," and of those, 358 are termed "major teaching hospitals." By definition, teaching hospitals are those in which there are approved residency teaching programs (combinations of classroom teaching with hands-on experience in caring for patients), as well as facilities for highly specialized (tertiary) patient care and for biomedical research. *Major* teaching hospitals are those that sponsor or participate in at least four approved residency programs, with at least two programs from the following six: family practice, internal medicine, obstetrics/gynecology, pediatrics, psychiatry, and surgery.

In 1989, there were 358 major teaching hospitals associated with our 127 U.S. medical schools, all of which met the qualifications of membership in COTH. They varied greatly in bed capacity; more than half (183) had more than 500 beds, in contrast to the 2,508 non-teaching hospitals that had fewer than 100 beds. Most (132) of the COTH members were located in the Northeast. Seventy-four were owned by municipalities, counties, and states, 54 by churches, and 4 by for-profit organizations. Although COTH hospitals made up only 6.4% of all U.S. hospitals, they employed 29% of the registered nurses, and had 79% of the entire residency population of the United States and 61% of its salaried MDs and dentists. COTH hospitals contained 21% of the 958,459 beds in U.S. hospitals, and accounted for 23% of the 31 million hospital admissions and 28% of the 245 million outpatient visits. The charity costs of COTH hospitals were five times larger than those of all non-teaching hospitals.

In 1987, teaching hospital costs on a per admission basis were 56% higher than those of non-teaching hospitals. Contributing to these higher costs were the educational costs for supervision and training of all residents, plus the service costs to sicker patients for the highly specialized procedures available in major teaching hospitals, plus the research costs not fully compensated for by externally funded research grants. Until now, these higher costs have been justified by the belief that, in the long term, the public will be better served by the high-quality professional health personnel trained in these major teaching hospitals. In the past, these higher costs were met by third-party payers (Medicare, Medicaid, and all other insurers) in a process called "cross-subsidization." Today, however, there is increasing concern that cross-subsidies will soon be greatly curtailed as insurers enforce increasingly stringent cost-containment measures. These economies are likely to fall most heavily on the elderly, who are making up ever larger proportions of the total population and of all hospital admissions, and on the teaching hospitals to which almost all of the uninsured turn for care.

AHCs, by definition, include a medical school, a major teaching hospital, and at least one other health education program, such as nursing, dentistry, or pharmacy, and any of some 25 other training programs in allied health skills such as medical technician, physical therapist, audiologist, and emergency technician. AHCs vary enormously in size, however it is measured: number of employed personnel, number of students, number of beds, annual operating budgets, number of teaching hospitals, number of educational programs. For instance, among the 123 AHCs extant in 1989, the number of schools and full-scale educational programs varied from 2 to 8 and the number of major teaching hospitals from 1 to 19. But, to the best of my knowledge, there has been no compilation of other parameters of size and activity (such as research intensity or operating budget), even though each institution surely keeps track of such descriptors in order to defend its costs to insurers and to its parent university.

The Association of Academic Health Centers (AAHC), incorporated in 1968, represents 100 institutions (5 in Canada). It provides a forum for the interchange of information among its members, who participate in public debates on health service issues and react to formulations of national health policy—i.e., who act as a lobby (*AAHC Directory*, 1989). Member institutions are represented in the AAHC by senior health administration officers (such as chancellors, presidents, or vice-presidents for health affairs). Those representatives meet annually, but the organization has no publications or journals, and it lacks a sophisticated database such as the Institutional Profile System of the AAMC that services the U.S. medical schools.

An AHC is big business. The most appealing aspects of such an enterprise are 24-hour availability of routine as well as specialized medical care to the community and referrals from a much wider area; a social institution serving persons from all economic and social backgrounds; a training center for young professionals exposed to a broad array of medical and social problems; and a research center with a wide variety of scientific skills and disciplines.

But the down side of AHCs is becoming increasingly apparent and deeply troubling to many highly qualified observers. For instance, as service responsibilities increase in number and complexity, the full-time clinical staff of the medical school is spread more thinly in its relationships with undergraduate medical students and residents. As a result, the teaching of students is increasingly performed by residents with only 3 or 4 years' postgraduate experience. The chairmen of the medical schools' clinical departments are by definition the chiefs of the hospitals' clinical services, with loyalties split between the two institutional entities—school and hospital. The concentration of highly technological procedures and appliances in an AHC promotes an overgrowth of subspecialties, which in turn leads subspecialists to concentrate increasingly on procedure-driven income generation. The perceived need for income to pay young clinical staff members focuses the attention of the medical staff on a rapidly changing population of in-patients with complicated illnesses, rather than on out-patients who are less sick. (Ambulatory medicine is less productive of income, but it offers a far better cross section of the medical problems faced daily by physicians in practice.) And as AHCs grow in size by merging with nearby community hospitals, the teaching of medical students and residents is increasingly weakened through dilution of the time and personal mentoring of experienced supervisors. Thus, the collegiality of the formerly smaller, closer-knit medical school has visibly decreased—to the detriment of all participants, in the view of many observers.

The mergers and acquisitions of Wall Street were long antedated by those that have made the teaching hospitals of medical schools into the behemoths we recognize as AHCs. The need for money has made the AHCs increasingly dependent on third-party payers and other pre-payment systems, obscuring the primary educational mission of the medical school. Harvey (1968) called for divorce of the service function from the education/research function of the medical school; later observers have echoed this plea vigorously and convincingly in their eagerness to see teaching re-established as the primary focus of the medical school—with better teaching by teachers better rewarded for their more personal attention to the educational needs and social maturation of their students. The emphasis on research that peaked in the late 1960s distracted the clinical faculties from teaching, and publications as a measure of research productivity came to be the yardstick by which all staff members were judged to be worthy of promotion and tenure. But the economic problems of the 1980s caused clinical departments to escalate in size—not to teach, not to perform research, but to generate the service income on which the clinical departments depend for survival. In today's AHCs, service more than pays its own way; research comes close to self-support; but teaching is an activity that has no easily characterized product for which a superb teacher can be appropriately judged and rewarded. Clearly, there is a growing imbalance among the three missions of U.S. medical schools, an imbalance created in earlier years by the perceived need for research productivity to enrich the intellectual atmosphere of the school, and more recently by the need for income that has led to the formation and growth of AHCs.

Medical schools have allowed their independence to be eroded as they turned to external sources for research funding. The major source of this external funding is the NIH, which is the subject of a later chapter.

This is why business has made inroads

SUMMARY AND CONCLUSIONS

The number of active physicians in the United States has risen from 300,000 in 1969 to 537,000, of whom 92% have consistently been engaged in the practice of medicine. Since 1958, the number of U.S. medical schools has risen from 72 to 127 and the number of graduates has risen fourfold, to more than 16,000 per year since 1925. Applicants to medical schools have varied widely in number, exceeding the capacity of U.S. schools to admit them by as much as 200% in 1950; at present, the ratio of applicants to matriculants has fallen to 1.6 to 1. Anecdotal perceptions aside, there is as yet no hard evidence of a decline in their scholastic aptitude, but there is a striking decrease in the number of college students majoring in the life sciences. This is an alarming trend, because this is the main pool from which medical school applicants are drawn.

Full-time faculty members of U.S. medical schools have increased in number even more rapidly than the total number of medical students, a fivefold increase since 1960. The major cause of this increase, which has occurred mainly in the clinical departments (medicine, surgery, pediatrics, etc.), is the pressing need in U.S. medical schools for income generation through service to patients. Service income has become the major source of support in U.S. medical schools (45%), almost double that from all government sources, while endowment income amounts to only 2% of the total income. Although tuition and fees to U.S. medical schools make up less than 8% of their total income, the cost of tuition to students has risen fourfold since 1960, and large-scale indebtedness is now a serious burden on more than half of all students.

The number of accredited hospitals in the United States is about 5,600, of which 358 are major teaching hospitals attached to medical schools, each with multiple residency training programs and paramedical training schools. Mainly because the money for teaching and residents' salaries comes from general hospital funds, the cost per patient admission is considerably higher there than in non-teaching hospitals; this will be a prime target for cost cutting in the future by Medicare and the private insurance industry. As AHCs have increasingly become big business, the quality of teaching, and the collegiality and personal autonomy that academic doctors enjoyed in the past, have markedly declined.

The general health of the public has certainly improved due to the increasing sophistication of medical management and access to better medical care over the last 40 years, even though at least 15% of the population is under-insured and has little access to these advantages. As a career, however, medicine has become much less attractive to college students, and academic medicine has suffered even more serious setbacks as a consequence of the demands for income generation and the resultant depersonalization of care and diminished collegiality within the largest and richest AHCs.

3

What Is Clinical Research?

THE CONCEPT OF RESEARCH

In the broadest sense of the word, research as a human endeavor began with Genesis. Walter Bradford Cannon, the eminent Harvard physiologist, said in 1945: "in spite of the testimony that it was curiosity which lost us Paradise, I am sure that all who are aware of the fruits of the Tree of Knowledge would agree that they have become abundant because of the spying and trying of inquisitive scientists." Curiosity certainly is at the root of every kind of research— the desire to know why and how, as well as what.

The word "research" itself has an interesting derivation. It comes from the French verb *chercher* (to search) from Late Latin *circare,* which the *Encyclopedia Britannica* translates as "to go round in a circle"; researchers know how true that can be! Peyton Rous, whose discovery of a viral cause for cancer in chickens at 31 years of age was rewarded with a Nobel Prize at 87, was fond of distinguishing REsearch from reSEARCH: the former indicating an activity of repeated searching in a pedestrian manner, the latter signifying discovery. Alan Gregg (1941) distinguished going back *of* the evidence from going back *to* the evidence. The *Oxford English Dictionary* clearly distinguishes the two pronunciations and defines reSEARCH as "a search or investigation directed to the discovery of some fact by careful consideration or study of a subject." The *Encyclopedia Britannica* is even more specific, characterizing it as "inquiry directed to the discovery of truth, and in particular the trained scientific investigation of the principles and facts of any subject, based on original and first-hand study of authorities or experiment." Rous would smilingly have labeled the subordinate staff writers of *Time* magazine REsearchers, certain that he and his scientific colleagues at the Rockefeller Institute for Medical Research were reSEARCHERS.

The word "research" is used today in so many ways by so many different kinds of people that each of us accepts the word without thinking exactly what we mean by it. In 1941 Alan Gregg reported a deeply insightful essay entitled "Medical Research Described," with lucid paragraphs on what research is *not;*

Researcher ≠ Experimenter

and W. I. B. Beveridge, whose delightful primer for beginners in scientific investigation has been favorite reading since 1951, noted: "Research is one of those highly complex and subtle activities that usually remain quite unformulated in the minds of those who practice [it]. This is probably why most scientists think that it is not possible to give any formal instruction in how to do research."

Every commentator agrees that the obligatory first step is observation: the process of looking and seeing something from as many angles as possible, and deciding how to describe the entity so precisely that others can appreciate fully what is being observed. Fitting an observation into one's past experience—making sense of it—may be the next step in a process that occurs even in animals. What appears to be uniquely human is the capacity to take a third step: devising a hypothesis to explain the observation—and finally, a fourth step—testing that hypothesis by experimentation. Of course, that last step may not be immediately possible. Einstein waited many years before certain astronomical events allowed scientists to test his theory of relativity. Einstein was certainly a researcher, even if not an experimenter.

Which inquiries deserve to be dignified by the term "research" is not easy to decide. That may be why there has been no definitive study of the evolution of the research process by scientists or scientist-historians. Supreme Court Justice Potter Stewart's widely accepted description of pornography ("I can't really define it, but I know it when I see it") may have to suffice here.

As we approach the subject of this chapter, clinical research, consider next the word "biomedical." Here is a word of fairly recent coinage, presumably an amalgam of "biological" and "medical." The merged word was first used in a foreword written by Arno B. Luckhardt to a book on the evolution of scientific English by Edmund Andrews in 1947 (but the word itself did not appear in the text of the book). It seems to have come into common usage after World War II in connection with atomic bomb testing in the Pacific, where biologists and physicians were deeply engaged in studies of the biologic effects of radiation on experimental animals. The earliest *official* use of the term appears to have been the 1949 designation of George LeRoy as director of the Biomedical Division of Operation Greenhouse, the atomic bomb testing program in the Marshall Islands in 1951. "Biomedical" does *not* appear in the records of earlier military and civilian groups engaged in radiation research: Operation Crossroads, The Joint Commission for Investigation of Effects of the Atomic Bomb in Japan, or the Manhattan Project.

"Biomedical" as a term was preceded by "biophysics," coined by Karl Pearson in 1892 (*Oxford English Dictionary,* 1989), and "biochemistry," first used by Hoppe-Seyler in 1877 and firmly established by Hofmeister in 1901 (Kohler, 1973). At any rate, and wherever the term arose, "biomedical" is the inclusive word today for the many kinds of research funded by the NIH and performed in our medical schools and medical research institutes by MDs, MD-PhDs, PhDs, and others, and whose content runs the gamut from strictly biological to strictly clinical.

BASIC RESEARCH AND APPLIED RESEARCH

Consider next two parlous words in the scientific lexicon: "basic" and "applied." For many in science, "basic" confers the cachet of knowledge pursued for its own sake, with no practical goal in mind. In contrast, "applied" is a term that suggests utility, market value, and the down-to-earth translation of useless into useful science. These two terms, when used thoughtfully, are perfectly acceptable descriptors of two kinds of research activity. However, all too often there is a pejorative connotation: basic is superior, applied inferior. That implication of first- and second-ratedness I find to be so offensive that I have tried in this book not to use these terms at all if I can find an acceptable substitute.

Many authors have written in fervent defense of *basic research,* driven by pressures inside and outside government to spend taxpayers' dollars more directly for the benefit of the public. This defense has required that terms be precisely defined. In 1959 Charles V. Kidd, writing from the NIH director's office, discussed the confusion about the meaning of the term by federal authorities disbursing and university officials receiving funds for so-called basic research. Kidd, speaking from the viewpoint of the disbursers, noted two contrasting definitions: one, "investigator-centered," speaks of investigators' motives and intentions and the freedom with which they work; the other, "substance-centered," focuses on the research product—its breadth of significance and generalizability, rather than the investigator's freedom to pursue whatever he desires to know and understand. Kidd concluded that neither definition was entirely adequate or informative for Congress, for the public, or for the federal administrators guiding the disbursement of grant funds. He concluded that, in his best reconciliation of terms, "a plea that the Federal Government 'support more basic research' is a plea for administration of a larger proportion of federal research funds in a manner which places few restrictions upon investigators."

In considering how best to distinguish basic from applied research, I found two definitions of basic research that I think are understandable, useful, and highly acceptable; both appeared in 1976. In their often-quoted analysis of the origins of great advances in the diagnosis and treatment of cardiopulmonary diseases, Comroe and Dripps described research as basic "when the investigator, in addition to observing, describing and measuring, attempts to determine *mechanisms responsible for the observed effects* [emphasis mine]; with our definition, basic research can be on healthy or sick people, on animals, tissues, cells, or subcellular components."

In the same year, the President's Biomedical Research Panel (chairman: Lewis Thomas) warned against the commonly held view that "at one extreme basic science is a purposeless, almost random activity in which the search for useful or usable *information* is obtained, while at the other extreme applied science is seen as exclusively concerned with *products* ready for marketing [emphasis mine]. Others believe [and the panel clearly disagreed] that applied science is whatever is done in connection with human beings and their diseases, while basic is the term for all the rest."

The panel went on to say, "We suggest that basic and applied science differ in their relative degrees of *certainty and uncertainty.*" "It is characteristic of basic research as a primarily *exploring* activity that it must be done in an atmosphere of some uncertainty." The investigator who designs his experiments well "can proceed with confidence that he will get answers, but since he is working in unknown territory he cannot have certainty as to the nature of those answers"; "his mind must be kept open to surprises." Looking at these issues from a sociologist's viewpoint, Merton (1985) noted that basic research adds to the intellectual capital that comprises scientific knowledge, whereas "applied research draws on that capital to arrive at new methods of achieving practical objectives that are themselves outside the sphere of basic knowledge."

The Thomas panel went on to say that "applied science is done quite differently, under the influence of a necessarily high degree of certainty," which ensures that "the outcome can be predicted." They cited as an example in the clinical field "the experiments of largest scale and complexity [what are called today "controlled clinical trials"], collaborative tests for new therapeutic or diagnostic agents in human subjects." The panel also warned that "the methods employed for planning and executing the two kinds of research are radically different": basic research puts demands on the imagination of the investigator and "his capacity to change his mind and his approach, when new developments occur." "Applied science requires that the work be laid out sequentially on carefully arranged time schedules—[and] the protocol for the experiment, once launched, cannot be changed on individual whim." Thus, the panel concluded that it is "an urgent matter to be sure that one approach is not misapplied to the other sort of problem—if the planning and tight organization schedules of applied science are misapplied to problems of high uncertainty, it will not turn out well."

Clearly, these two 1976 definitions say much the same thing, but in different words: it is the nature of the question asked and the manner in which an answer is sought that characterize basic research. It is not the doctoral degree of the researcher, or the name of the department in which that person performs the research, or the object under study, be it a marine animal, a leafy tree, or a human being.

Accordingly, it is misleading to call the non-clinical departments of a medical school faculty the *basic* departments, for this implies that the clinical departments are capable only of performing applied, targeted, or utilitarian research. In fact, basic research, as defined above, is performed in both of these divisions of the faculty, and so is applied research. Therefore, I have chosen in this book to speak of the "pre-clinical" and "clinical" departments. The latter are much engaged in studies on and service to patients, while the former are not.

In our medical schools, the primary mission of pre-clinical departments (such as anatomy, pathology, pharmacology, microbiology, physiology, biochemistry, and molecular biology) is teaching; their secondary mission, conducting research, may or may not be basic in nature. By the same token, clinicians in medicine, surgery, pediatrics, neurology, psychiatry (and their many subspecialties) are concerned, first and foremost, with patients and with teaching their students and residents how to recognize and cope with disease, but the research they carry out can be (but often is not) as basic in nature as that performed by the pre-clinical groups.

To illustrate, consider a study that asks how a given drug performs its functions in a given situation, why it works the way it does, and how it is disposed of. These are searching questions posed without foreknowledge of the results that can only be obtained through experimentation, and they deserve to be called "basic." In contrast, if the study is designed to compare the safety and efficacy of a new drug with the safety and efficacy of one already accepted in practice, I would call this applied and not basic research. Such trials, however essential they may be to progress in clinical practice, usually do not contribute to a deeper understanding of a fundamental biologic question. Indeed, we can say that because such trials are highly protocolized, they are performed in an atmosphere of certainty; a "yes" or "no" answer is inevitable if the study is well designed (and useless if it is not). In this sense, the large-scale, controlled clinical trials of new drugs and new technologies are examples of applied and not basic research. However essential the results obtained, rarely do such studies lead to deeper understandings of human biology.

CLINICAL RESEARCH

We come, at last, to clinical research, the primary focus of this book. Comroe and Dripps (1976) wrote: "We define research as clinically oriented, even if it is performed entirely on animals, tissues, cells, or sub-cellular particles, *if the author mentions even briefly* [emphasis mine] an interest in the diagnosis, treatment, or prevention of a clinical disorder, or in explaining the basic [did they not mean underlying?] mechanisms of a sign or symptom of the disease itself." If the author has *not* given evidence that his research was prompted by questions dealing with the nature of disease or the mechanisms of disease phenomena, I consider that research to be non-clinical even when it is performed by MDs in a medical school environment.

I will show in the following pages why, in analyzing the published reports of scientific studies, it is useful to distinguish non-clinical from clinical research and, further, to subdivide clinical research itself into several categories. I will then illustrate each of these sub-types and rationalize the categorization process.

But, first, I must return to an earlier leitmotif and speak about clinical REsearch (as distinct from clinical reSEARCH). Our medical and scientific journals contain two sorts of articles that are extremely useful to readers but are really not reSEARCH at all because they do not originate in a research question— namely, reviews and case reports. Reviews of the literature on a given topic pull together what has been accomplished worldwide over the years; they are most useful when the author attempts a critical evaluation of those studies. A second kind of review gathers together what clinicians at a given institution have learned or observed about the diagnosis or treatment of a particular human disorder; this is done through a survey of the hospital records of that subset of patients. In neither case does the review-writer require the facilities of a laboratory, but rather those of a library or of a hospital record room. In fact, the reviewer has little or no control over the subject matter (except for its analysis and presentation), since by definition the review is retrospective; the reviewer is simply a recorder or analyst of past events. The author's motivation is to summarize what has been learned or observed. In both cases, the effort is useful and instructive for the author as well as for the reader, but it is not reSEARCH. (Gregg said this pithily: "Summarizing or compiling facts is not research.")

Many case reports published in medical journals describe an interesting new manifestation or newly recognized illness in one or a small number of patients; they are useful in alerting the medical profession to the recognition of a new clinical entity. Case reports are descriptive and characteristically opportunistic, testifying to the acute powers of observation of the author; they are certainly clinical, but I cannot call them reSEARCH. In my analysis of the publication output of clinical scientists, I have customarily distinguished an author's case reports from his research reports in order to assess the interests and activities of that person at a given time in his career. But because of the non-experimental nature of case reports, I have chosen not to classify them as any kind of research, regardless of their intrinsic value and interest for readers.

Clinical reSEARCH has a number of synonyms: "clinical science," "experimental medicine," "medical science," and "clinical investigation"; all are very broad general terms that mean the same thing. The scientific periodicals that employ such terms in their titles make available to their readers a wide variety of scientific pursuits that range from meticulous studies on small numbers of whole human beings, on the one hand, to general descriptions of health and disease in large populations, on the other: from purely descriptive to intensely manipulative studies; from purely bedside observations to bench research on "scraps and fragments" of people (J.B.S. Haldane's phrase); from the study of animal models of human biology to computer-modeling of physiologic processes; and from comparisons of new with old treatment methods to assessments of treatment outcomes in social and economic terms.

I have found that these widely varied research activities—all of which require special training, facilities, and funding, and all of which are properly called clinical ReSEARCH—can be divided into seven types or categories. For these purposes, I have refined an earlier taxonomic design of Bever (1980, in collaboration with Richard Landau) and expanded it by adding one further category. In the next chapter, I define the characteristics of each of the seven categories and give examples from my own research experience in each category.

My aim in describing the vast terrain of clinical research in terms of its components is to attempt to find a way to measure changes over time in the attention paid to each activity by researchers and by funding agencies. (I cannot say too strongly that the division of clinical research into seven categories implies no value judgments of their relative merits.) The results I have obtained in analyzing the clinical research literature in these terms are described in Chapters 5 and 8; I believe they will show that the pursuit of each of these research "disciplines" calls on different sets of training skills, technical facilities, and methods of thinking.

SUMMARY AND CONCLUSIONS

"Clinical research," a commonly used term, is synonymous with "experimental medicine," "clinical science," and "clinical investigation." As an activity, it now encompasses much more than "bedside research," as was once the case (the word "clinical" comes from *klinikos,* Greek for a physician who attends bedridden patients). "Research" itself has come into common usage in science only in this century, in the sense of exploration, discovery, and careful study of unexplained phenomena. But in the vernacular, research has come to mean almost any sort of "looking things up," as in reference libraries, dictionaries, or *Who's Who.* The suggestion has been made that these two meanings be distinguished by accenting the second syllable when scientific exploration is meant (reSEARCH), and the first (REsearch) when the activity is merely one of looking up facts and figures in texts and reference books.

"Biomedical" is of very recent origin. This term, linking "biological" and "medical," was apparently first coined in 1947 to describe the many kinds of studies undertaken by various kinds of scientists in defining the biological effects of radiation in atomic bomb tests in the Pacific after World War II. The word biomedical is a useful adjective that describes the many kinds of research so generously funded by the federal government and by private sources that aim at gaining clearer understandings of biologic phenomena in all species, including human beings.

"Basic" and "applied" are terms that too often are used pejoratively in common parlance. A plea is made in this chapter for restricting the term "basic research" to those investigations undertaken in a spirit of uncertainty, where the exploratory nature of a study is implicit and its outcome is not predictable. What many call *basic science departments* in U.S. medical schools (such as biochemistry and molecular biology) are more appropriately named "pre-clinical departments," since basic research (undertaken in uncertainty) is just as much the purview of faculty members in the clinical as in the pre-clinical departments.

This attention to terminology and definitions leads in the next chapter to a dissection of clinical research into seven categories, each different in scope, background training, and facilities, but all complementary and essential for the pursuit of progress in medicine.

4

Seven Categories of Clinical Research

The activity called clinical research in Chapter 3 describes a vast terrain of different objectives, skills, funding, and technical facilities. It has proven useful to divide this terrain into seven parts as a means of measuring changes over time in the attention paid to each of those component parts by researchers and by agencies.

1. *Studies of Mechanisms in Human Disease*

   This consists of studies in which the investigator seeks to refine current characterizations of disease processes (or health) and to explore unresolved questions in human biology by controlled observations or manipulations (or both) of patients or volunteers and their environments (such extrinsic factors as diet, exercise, sleep, study setting, stress, drugs, etc.). Pharmacokinetic studies belong in this category. These various kinds of mechanistic studies require the special facilities of a clinical research center with dedicated in-patient or out-patient areas (or both) and trained support staffing. The responsible investigator may or may not have performed the required laboratory work personally, but he *does* have control over both the benchwork and the clinical aspects of such studies.

   Example: metabolic studies of volunteers on diets rich in palmitic vs. stearic acid in relation to changes in plasma lipids and lipoproteins; pharmacologic studies on the mode of action of a plasma-lipid-lowering drug in patients with hypercholesterolemia.

2. *Studies of Management of Disease*

   This consists of studies in which the investigator, working directly with patients or volunteers, prospectively conducts controlled observations on an incompletely tested new diagnostic or therapeutic technique or device, often in comparison with an accepted one. This category also encompasses tests of preventive measures, all drug studies aimed at establishing safety and efficacy, and studies of patient-compliance, since all are directly relevant to management of disease.

   Example: a large-scale, controlled clinical trial of a drug in relation to the incidence of new events of coronary heart disease.

3. *In Vitro Studies on Materials of Human Origin*
   These studies are conducted in relation to a stated or strongly implied clinical issue in which the patients or volunteers providing such materials as blood, tissues, or excreta are *not* directly managed or experimentally manipulated by the laboratory investigator who works on those materials. Human genome studies fall into this category, as do the research results of autopsy and surgical pathology studies.

Example: definition of receptor defects in fibroblasts derived from skin biopsy specimens of patients with familial hypercholesterolemia, and their genetic determinants.

4. *Animal Models of Human Health or Disease*
   Here the investigator explores some aspect of human physiology or clinical disease through studies performed in animals (sometimes in mathematical or computer models) by means of experimental manipulations, usually prospectively.

Example: studies in non-human primates of the regression of arteriosclerotic lesions produced by dietary manipulations.

5. *Field Surveys*
   Here the investigator or teams of investigators search for risk factors for human disease in open population groups, either descriptively or through active manipulations (epidemiologic studies). The kindred studies of geneticists fall into this category, as do psychological surveys aimed at refinements in understanding of clinical issues or human behavior.

Example: the search in open populations for risk factors for coronary heart disease.

6. *Development of New Technologies*
   The *invention, development* and quality-control testing of new diagnostic and therapeutic methods (bioassays, scanning techniques, biostatistical methods, vaccines, etc.) in this category are clearly distinct from their *application* in management of disease (Category 2).

Example: studies attempting to define the optimal technical conditions under which arteriography can be used to measure changes in the size of arteriosclerotic lesions in major blood vessels

7. *Assessment of Health Care Delivery*
   In these studies, investigators examine the societal and economic consequences of health management practices, both old and new, or study the infrastructure of delivery systems (medical or allied health professional education, hospital or clinic administration, medico-legal studies, health insurance studies, geographic distribution of professional skills, health manpower needs, resource allocations). This field has come to be called "health sciences research."

Example: comparative evaluations of the efficacy of coronary bypass surgery in terms of costs and side effects in different treatment centers.

NON-CLINICAL RESEARCH

This very large body of biomedical research is best described as separate from the seven categories of clinical research. These studies are performed in such varied disciplines as chemistry, physics, biology, zoology, anatomy, biochemistry, and microbiology. While they contribute importantly to new understandings of biologic processes, they are not directly related to clinical issues and do not originate in stated or implied questions dealing with human health or disease.

DISTINCTIONS AMONG THE SEVEN CATEGORIES

Differences in Subject Matter

The distinctions between Categories 1, 2, 5, and 7 must be carefully drawn. I will illustrate by using examples drawn from my own research experience. In human beings fed diets rich in saturated fatty acids, the effects can be described in terms of changes in the concentration of circulating lipids and lipoproteins; or in terms of changes in clotting mechanisms, membrane permeability, or the rheologic qualities of blood: Such studies fall into Category 1 (mechanistic studies). The effects of dietary fat exchanges also can be defined in terms of vascular changes in high-risk males. This is a management-of-disease question (Category 2). Alternatively, the effects of such fat exchanges can be considered in terms of preventing the consequences of arteriosclerotic disease in large field studies of seemingly healthy population groups (Category 5). Finally, dietary manipulation can be studied from an economic and social point of view in terms of recommending such dietary changes to the population as a whole; this is research on health care delivery (Category 7).

Another example: comparative drug studies on the treatment of certain cancers (Category 2) are different from pharmacologic studies of the uptake and disposal of those drugs in human beings (Category 1). Both are essential, but they are differently motivated and differently undertaken.

From now on, I will speak of Category 1 research—i.e., mechanistic studies in patients or volunteers—as "Basic patient-oriented research (Basic POR)"—and of Category 2 research—i.e., studies on the management of disease—as "Applied POR." I will defend this usage later.

Differences in Strategies of Attack

These various research activities differ not only in their subject matter but also in the methods of thinking employed by their investigators—how to frame the question and how to tackle it. Certain research activities are exclusively reductionistic in approach, and others are integrative. For instance, in vitro studies on materials of human origin (Category 3) are reductionistic: the investigator seeks to eliminate as many experimental variables as possible in order to isolate the single variable of greatest interest. In contrast, most research in whole human beings (or animals, or population groups) is strongly integrative, and reductionistic only insofar as the laboratory techniques employed are rigidly controlled to eliminate undesirable variables. The complex nature of the biochemical and physiologic interplay that characterizes a whole organism prevents the investigator from focusing on one variable to the exclusion of the rest, for to overlook or even to minimize that complexity would be to destroy the wholeness (an example in clinical research of Heisenberg's uncertainty principle). W.B. Cannon (1945) spoke of himself as an integrative physiologist interested in the responses of the total organism, and in "a synthesis of the functioning of organs and systems of organs as they cooperate in the behavior of the organism as a whole."

The integrative investigator, in adapting to this interplay of variables, must have the skill to reach new biologic understandings despite the existence of uncontrolled variables. This approach demands a different mind set and training background from that of the reductionist. The integrative scientist is necessarily broadly based in physiology, biochemistry, and clinical medicine, but must also be knowledgeable in the laboratory skills required for application to the problem under study. Where the reductionist bores in more deeply (but narrowly), the integrationist travels a broader terrain.

Differences in Facilities and Training

The seven categories of clinical research also differ from each other in the technical facilities that each requires and in the training that makes the best use of those facilities. Basic POR researchers (Category 1) depend on a wide variety of ancillary personnel with special skills to help in the management of their patients (or volunteers), but also on the laboratory personnel they must train to make the best use of the techniques required by the investigation. Applied POR investigators dealing with research on the management of disease (Category 2) do not always require the precise controls afforded by a metabolic ward and diet kitchen; they can often manage adequately with out-patient facilities if supported by specially trained nurses, coordinators, and record managers. Researchers on animal models of human biologic processes (Category 4) require resources that are just as sophisticated as those needed in study of human beings, with the same attention to ethics and humaneness that apply in POR; but in addition, they must have a broad understanding of a wide variety of animal species and a special appreciation of the many subtle differences between inbred laboratory animals and outbred human beings. Field studies (Category 5) in large population groups of free-living citizens depend heavily on social service skills, and on visiting nurses, physician-assistants, and statisticians, but also critically on the supervision of leaders who are broadly based integrationists. The development of new technologies (Category 6) is the domain of clinical chemists, engineers, and technicians; they are inventors who must be compulsive about quality control. The scanning techniques rapidly being perfected today require the skills of mathematicians, physicists, radiologists, and biochemists working at many interfaces between reductionism and holism. And, finally, those engaged in research on health care assessment (Category 7) must be skilled clinicians working closely with social scientists, economists, lawyers, administrators, ethicists, and even politicians. Workers in this special domain seek to put the diagnostic and prognostics of internal medicine on a more quantitative base.

Despite these many differences (subject matter, strategies, training, and facilities), some investigators move from one category of research to another, perhaps simultaneously but more often over the long span of their careers. Indeed, there are no barriers among the seven categories, and their boundary lines are not always sharp. All are essential research activities, all are inter-related and inter-dependent, and all must be encouraged to prosper.

The progress of science depends on the continuing development of new methods, as well as on new intellectual insights and inspirations. Clinical research is not performed exclusively by medical graduates, nor is non-clinical research carried out exclusively by PhDs. Since the medical graduate has an unique understanding of and experience in human biology, it is not surprising that most case reports and reviews of hospital records are written by individuals with medical degrees. On the other hand, it is becoming increasingly apparent that more and more PhDs, with their concentrated training in physics, chemistry, and biology, have become interested in pursuing careers in clinical departments and in teaming up with MDs to undertake research on subjects of importance for human health. This trend deserves encouragement in every conceivable way.

Clearly, the pursuit of clinical research calls on a multitude of different training skills and personality types. These differences, as well as clear-cut differences in subject matter, justify the distinctions I have made in setting up the seven-category taxonomy. In later chapters, I will demonstrate the utility of these distinctions. But it must be re-emphasized that making any value judgments on the merits of one category of clinical research over another misses the crucial point: *all* categories are essential to progress in medical science, to the delivery of better care to the public, and eventually to the prevention of disease.

SOME REDEFINITIONS OF POR

It should be clear by now that POR is actually not one but two entities. Mechanistic studies (Category 1) and management of disease studies (Category 2) are both patient-oriented. Both require human beings as subjects of study and experimentation, but one is Basic POR and the other is Applied POR. These two terms, "basic" and "applied," "outlawed" earlier, must be re-instated and used in a clarifying, non-pejorative manner. Category 1 POR is better called "Basic" POR because it describes the kind of research that is undertaken in an atmosphere of uncertainty (the President's Biomedical Research Panel Report's definition of "basic" in 1976) and that focuses on testing hypotheses about some aspect of human biology that we do not yet fully understand (Comroe and Dripp's definition of "basic"). Category 2 POR is better called "Applied" POR because it is performed in the certainty that a clear-cut "yes" or "no" outcome will be revealed: for instance, a new diagnostic or therapeutic procedure will be found to be better or worse than one relied on before, or a new drug will prove to be more or less effective and safe than others in generally accepted use.

Applied POR, then, can often be performed in out-patient settings if patients do not require hospitalization, as in drug testing for prevention of a second heart attack in individuals who have already had one. Applied POR may also be carried out in a specialized treatment center like a neonatal unit, as in comparing phototherapy (a procedure) with tin (Sn^{4+})-protoporphyrin (a drug) for amelioration of neonatal jaundice: In this case, safety and efficacy must be ascertained and certified in potentially very sick infants.

By the same token, Basic POR may or may not require the specialized facilities available at the very large NIH Clinical Center in Bethesda or in the (presently) 78 much smaller general clinical research centers (GCRCs) throughout the United States. Studies on the absorption and disposition of drugs may be feasible in out-patient settings if the metabolism of those drugs is rapid and simple; but, if their turnover is complicated by passage through several pools and pathways, and if the end products must be measured in sweat, tears, blood, urine, or feces, then a clinical research center may be required. Thus, the high cost of clinical research centers can be justified by their dedication to experimental observations that cannot easily be performed elsewhere.

Studies performed outside such centers also can be either basic or applied, depending on the nature of the questions under test. Thus, it will come as no great surprise that the published results of POR do not always stem from studies performed in GCRC facilities. Although there are no hard data on the proportion of POR that demands GCRC facilities, a rather crude sampling procedure (to be described in Chapter 10) suggests that perhaps only one-third of Basic or Applied POR needs to be carried out in a GCRC.

I would make a strong argument for restricting the use of GCRCs *and* of the NIH Clinical Center to work that cannot be undertaken elsewhere. Indeed, studies that can be performed in general out-patient clinics without jeopardizing the validity of the findings should not take place in clinical research centers at all: These centers are too costly in terms of time, effort, and money to be so used.

The obverse of this statement is that clinical research centers should increasingly be devoted to mechanistic studies, to long-term themes or programs of research unfettered by protocols, to the kinds of explorations that cannot be performed elsewhere, and to the "fishing expeditions" that lead good investigators toward innovation and discovery. Observational and manipulative research demand time—often months—in groping for new insights. Indeed, time is the foremost asset of such clinical research centers—time in which all the clinical changes that occur can be observed and documented. Strong institutional support for Basic POR can best be expressed by protecting the time of its investigators through relieving them of many of the responsibilities demanded of non-research faculty members.

RECENT CHANGES IN BIOMEDICAL RESEARCH

Research Directions

Now that we have laid out a map on which the various domains of biomedical research have been identified and the boundaries among them drawn (loosely, and with no "trade barriers"), we can ask whether there has been any indication of "continental drift." Are non-clinical research and the seven categories of clinical research separate continents, with widely differing flora and fauna? Surely they are not, although the customs of the inhabitants of these "lands" differ widely, as do their tools and societal objectives.

When in simpler times the pursuit of scientific knowledge was undertaken by natural philosophers, the tools of science were few in number and low in precision, yet enormous strides were taken through observation and induction— in physics, astronomy, mathematics, and (considerably later) biology. The science of medicine got off to a very slow start, even after the shackles of ages-old dogma were thrown off in the sixteenth century by Paracelsus, who burned the texts of Galen in the city square of Basel in 1526. The methods applied up to the nineteenth century were more often observational than experimental until the introduction of physiologic experimentation by Beaumont in the 1820s and Bernard in the 1860s, in bacteriology by Pasteur and Koch, and in pathology by Virchow in the second half of the nineteenth century.

Clinical research, as we know it today, began with observation and description, and as methods were developed, it moved into experimentation and hypothesis testing. When a problem is approached from as many angles as the available methods allow, and when a solution is reached that fits with all the experimental observations, we say that we have reached a new truth—a truth that will remain unchallenged until newer and more powerful methodologic approaches or new intellectual insights are brought to bear on the matter and a more exact understanding is reached. Thus, the rate of progress toward new truths is governed by the introduction of new insights and new methods. Whichever comes first, the other necessarily follows.

In biomedical research after World War II, with abundant federal funding and institutional protection of time for research, there occurred a golden era in which great strides were taken simultaneously in human biology and laboratory science, with a product—molecular biology—that has revolutionized biomedical science. However, since the early and mid-1960s, federal funds have not matched the demands made on them; and since the mid-1970s, the time allowed for research has been increasingly eroded by institutional pressures, especially by the extraordinary increase in the need for income generation to keep solvent the bloated empires called "academic health centers (ACHs)." Thus, with less money for the support of increasingly sophisticated (and costly) facilities, and with less time to spend in exploring the research opportunities opened up by these new methods, it comes as no surprise that the earlier and less complex terrain of clinical research has changed, with the fragmentation of an earlier Gondwanaland into the several continents of non-clinical and clinical research.

It has been difficult to track these shifts except anecdotally. Lederberg (1982) spoke of three eras of clinical research: the first initiated by Koch's germ theory, the second characterized by signal advances in human physiology, and the current third era of molecular biology. Each of these eras was ushered in by innovations in methodology and new insights; but, even as the human genome becomes more fully mapped and our heredity better understood and described, there will remain large unexplored areas of human biology that represent the interplay of environmental forces and the human responses to them.

I know of only one previous attempt to quantify the changes in the terrain of biomedical research—that completed by Feinstein and his colleagues in 1967. They plotted the changes over the previous 12-year period in the research interests of three major clinical research societies in the United States—the Association of American Physicians, the American Society for Clinical Investigation, and the American Federation for Clinical Research. They did this by analyzing the abstracts submitted and programs presented annually at the three societies' joint meetings in Atlantic City, New Jersey. Feinstein et al. read some 7,000 abstracts and separated them into two broad categories—human and non-human—and into six subsets, depending on disease-, human-, and laboratory-orientation. Their analysis showed a marked decline in all human research and a striking rise in non-human, non-disease research. Thus, even during the golden era, a distinct turning away from clinical to non-clinical research was manifest in our most prestigious clincal investigation societies, a trend that has continued and indeed accelerated up to the present.

Feinstein's (1967) quantitative analyses of the predilections of clinical researchers shed little or no light on the *quality* of research performed by individual scientists, and indeed, I know of no perfect way to measure research quality. Each scientist develops his own standards of excellence in performing research and presenting it to others, either verbally or in writing. Some of us are casual about standards; others are driven by perfectionism. Each person's standards represent a combination of personality type with whatever has been learned through years of contacts with mentors and colleagues.

SUMMARY AND CONCLUSIONS

It is clarifying and useful to divide clinical research into seven categories of activity that differ from each other in their objectives, the means by which they are studied, the training and facilities that each requires.

Patient-oriented research (POR) is an integrative discipline. It copes with the complexity that is characteristic of whole organisms in order to understand the components of that complexity. Basic POR is the study of human beings (either patients or healthy volunteers) for the purpose of characterizing disease processes more precisely, and for gaining new insights into human responses to disturbances in chemical and behavioral makeup and to assaults by external factors. Thus, Basic POR is research on mechanisms, asking how and why certain phenomena occur in disease. In contrast, Applied POR is involved in management-of-disease questions, asking what is best, safest, and most useful among the drugs, vaccines, and procedures under test.

Laboratory studies on animal models of human disease are examples of reductionism in vivo, while studies of human materials, such as blood cells or skin growth under sterile culture conditions, exemplify reductionism in vitro: As variables are eliminated one by one, phenomena are described in finer and finer detail and then manipulated, but this ever-thinner "slice" becomes less and less representative of the whole from which it was derived.

In the last three decades, the focus of clinical investigators has shifted dramatically from integrative to reductionistic research. This is due largely to a fascination with the power of the new reductionist technologies of molecular biology to reach new insights at the molecular level and to do so rapidly. POR, on the other hand, is the most time-consuming form of clinical research, the most difficult, and the slowest. Thus, as physician-scientists have found themselves increasingly constrained in finding time for research, they have turned from POR to the reductionist modes of research.

5

Biomedical Research in the United States

We have looked at the nature of biomedical research and characterized the many different kinds of activities that are pursued by biomedical investigators, especially by clinical researchers. It is time now to ask, who are these investigators? How are they trained? How many are there? Where do they work? How are they supported? Later, we will consider in detail the objectives of the biomedical research system and its success in meeting those goals.

But first, we must deal with the size of the system and the origins of its practitioners. This task is greatly complicated by the fact that most researchers play multiple roles. This is particularly true of those with MD degrees, most of whom spend a great deal of time caring for patients, perhaps also teaching, and very likely in administrative activities as well.

According to the AMA Physician Masterfile (1990 edition), some 17,000 MDs claimed that research was their primary activity (see Chapter 2). There is no comparable tabulation of PhDs engaged primarily in research. The National Science Foundation's (NSF) annual tally of PhD scientists stated that some 45,000 (about half of all PhDs engaged in biomedical and medical sciences) were employed in R&D, but how many of these were active primarily in R as distinct from D is not known. The NSF data on PhDs are shown in Table 5–1, but the R question remains unanswered.

Another approach to the question of the current pool size of biomedical researchers in the United States is afforded by an in-house analysis of principal investigators (PIs) on NIH/ADAMHA grants and contracts in FY 1987 carried out for the NIH director by Sherman (1989). Those data (Table 5–2) show a total number of some 12,000 PIs, 45% of whom were MDs or MD-PhDs and 53% PhDs (and 2% other degree holders, not shown). This estimate of the total biomedical research pool (12,000) can validly be considered a minimum number for the United States, since it overlooks all researchers who were not PIs and all who carried out their research at sites other than U.S. medical schools.

Still another estimate is afforded by a study of some 10,000 full-time members of all U.S. departments of medicine in 1983, reported in 1987 by Gentile et al. This report, which will be described in more detail later, indicated that for this particular faculty group, 17 faculty members received research funding, but *not* as PIs on NIH grants and contracts, for every 10 members who *were* PIs, a ratio of 1.7 to 1. Thus, by combining the Sherman and Gentile analyses, it is reasonable to calculate that, for departments of medicine alone, there may have

Table 5-1 Number of PhDs Engaged in the Biological and Medical Sciences in the United States (1987)

Field and Type of Employer	Total Employed[a]	Colleges and Universities[b]	Hospitals and Clinics	Nonprofit Organizations[c]	Federal Gov't[d]	Industry[e]
Total employed	91,582	56,084	4,228	3,874	6,496	16,573
R&D	45,329	28,511	1,243	2,402	4,306	7,084
Professional services	6,501	2,445	1,670	137	29	1,914
Management and administration	12,781	4,845	606	867	1,619	3,600
Teaching	19,332	17,110	72	98	58	181
All others	7,639					

[a]Ph.D. degrees granted over the 42-year period 1944–86.
[b]Exclusive of 2-year colleges and lower-level schools.
[c]Foundations, think tanks, and affiliated laboratories.
[d]Exclusive of military, commissioned corps, state and local governments.
[e]Includes self-employed persons.

Source: NSF, *Characteristics of Doctoral Scientists and Engineers in the United States: 1987* (Pub. No. 88-331), Table 12, p. 32.

Table 5–2 Principal Investigators on NIH/ADAMHA Grants and Contracts in FY 1987

	All Degrees	Degrees Held		
		MDs Only	MD-PhDs Only	PhDs Only
All Departments				
Total faculty[a]	60,534	36,881	3,319	16,777
Number of PIs	12,003	4,406	965	6,390
Percent of all PIs with various degrees	100%	36.7	8.0	53.2
Pre-Clinical Departments				
Total faculty	11,960	2,143	694	8,703
Number of PIs	5,045	507	317	4,154
Percent who are PIs	42.2	23.7	45.7	47.7
Clinical Departments				
Total faculty	46,969	34,449	2,589	7,327
Number of PIs	6,596	3,829	629	1,927
Percent who are PIs	14.0	11.1	24.3	26.9
Other Academic Assignments				
Total positions	1,605	289	36	747
Number of PIs	362	70	19	264
Percent who are PIs	22.6	24.2	52.8	35.3

[a]Full-time faculty members in 127 U.S. medical schools.

Source: Charles R. Sherman, Office of the Director, NIH, summary report, May 1, 1989.

been as many as 7,300 biomedical researchers (2,700 PIs and 4,600 non-PIs with MD or PhD degrees). If it were warranted to extrapolate these medical department data to U.S. medical faculties as a whole (which is not easy to defend), we would reach a total of some 32,000 biomedical researchers in medical schools alone.

It would appear, then, that the number of biomedical researchers in U.S. medical schools alone lies somewhere between 12,000 and 32,000. The smaller number (the Sherman data) does not include all those who were supported by funding sources *other than* the NIH, and the larger number (the Gentile data) is suspect because it was derived from a self-administered questionnaire that surveyed only one of many medical school departments. At best this estimate includes both MDs and PhDs, and at worst it is based on a number of unwarranted assumptions, but it is the closest approximation to pool size that the available data permit.

MEDICINE: THE MAJOR DEPARTMENT IN U.S. MEDICAL SCHOOLS

The Sherman (1989) report showed the dominance of departments of medicine in U.S. medical schools in terms of faculty size and ability to win NIH grants as PIs. His data, abbreviated in Table 5–3, show that in 1987 the clinical faculties

Table 5–3   Dominant Clinical and Pre-Clinical Departments Among Full-Time
Faculties of All U.S. Medical Schools in FY1987[a]

	Full-Time Faculty Members			
	In All Clinical Depts.	In All Depts. of Med.	In All Pre-Clinical Depts.	In All Depts. of Biochem.
Total Number	46,969	13,448	11,960	1,958
As a percentage of the entire faculty	77.6%	22.2%	19.8%	3.2%
As a percentage of all clinical (or pre-clinical) faculties	100%	28.6%	100%	16.3%
Principal Investigators				
Total number	6,596	2,682	5,045	1,121
As a percentage of all PIs in their respective clinical (or pre-clinical) faculties	100%	40.4%	100%	22.2%

[a]Based on data in the AAMC Faculty Roster System (but exclusive of 1,605 individuals in assignments other than clinical and pre-clinical departments), linked with the number of PIs on NIH/ADAMHA grants and NIH contracts in the IMPAC database of the Division of Research Grants (DRG) of NIH, as compiled by Charles R. Sherman, Office of the Director, NIH, May 1, 1989.

outnumbered the pre-clinical faculties by nearly 4 to 1, that the department of medicine was the largest clinical department (29% of the entire clinical faculty), and that investigators in medicine won the lion's share of NIH grants as PIs (40% of all clinical faculty PIs). Clearly, full-time faculty members in departments of medicine must be regarded as major players in current biomedical research.

The Gentile (AAMC) report aimed at defining the "active investigator" by looking at individual members in all departments of medicine in 123 U.S. medical schools in 1983: their number, work habits, and research funding. The number of faculty members in medicine (all degrees) was 11,293; although responses to the AAMC questionnaire numbered only 7,947 (70%), the sample was found not to be biased in terms of age, sex, ethnic background, degree, or institution type (public or private). Gentile counted MDs, MD-PhDs, PhDs, and "other degrees" separately, tallied the number of NIH PIs in these degree categories, and related the research effort of the individual respondents to the research intensity of their respective schools. The study concluded by defining the active investigator in four operational terms: expenditure of at least 20% of working time in research, attraction of external funding, possession of dedicated laboratory space, and publication of at least one original research article in the 2-year period 1981–83. Only 37% of the respondents met all four criteria, and about half of these were NIH PIs. About half of the respondents spent less than 20%

of their time in research. In contrast, those devoting more than 40% of their time to research were as follows: MDs, 29.5%; MD-PhDs, 45.3%; and PhDs, 85.9%. Almost 30% of the MDs spent no time at all in research compared to 6.5% of the PhDs.

A revealing tally of research funding in the Gentile report (not tabulated here) indicated that of 7,147 faculty members holding MD or PhD degrees, 2,380 (33%) received no funds for research at all, 2,506 (35%) received NIH funding (and of these, 1,753 were NIH PIs), and 2,261 (32%) had funding from sources other than the NIH. Thus, for every 10 NIH PIs, there were 17 other researchers who were funded in some manner, but not as NIH PIs.

The nature of the research work performed by these members of the departments of medicine—whether it was non-clinical or fell into one of the seven categories of clinical research—was not explored in this survey (nor has this type of inquiry been made in any medical school survey, to my knowledge). For this reason, I undertook an independent analysis of the publications of some 900 members of three major clinical departments in order to determine not what faculty members say they do but rather the nature of the research they actually accomplish and publish.

A SURVEY OF THE RESEARCH PRODUCTIVITY OF MDs IN U.S. MEDICAL SCHOOLS

In 1988 I designed a study, with the help of Dr. Paul Jolly (AAMC), to evaluate changes in the research output—i.e., research publications—of three major clinical departments (medicine, pediatrics, and neurology) in three target years, 1977, 1982, and 1987. The way in which this survey (referred to later as the 3-D Survey) was performed (as well as others that will be presented later) is described in an appendix to this chapter: random sampling, tests of representativeness of the sampling, selection of research articles (as distinct from non-research reports) from the National Medical Library's (NML) Medline system, and categorizing them into one of the seven categories of clinical research (or, alternatively, designating them as non-clinical research).

The results of the 3-D Survey have been analyzed in several ways: in terms of the separate departmental publication outputs; in terms of individual faculty members and their publication of the various kinds of research; and in terms of changes over time through the most recent 10-year period. Statistical tests of significance were carried out by Dr. Anne Zeleniuch-Jacquotte, NYU Medical School, Institute of Environmental Medicine; proportions were compared using the binomial test or McNemar's test. The chi square for linearity was used to assess changes over time in proportions. Regression analysis was used to assess the time trends in the number of publications per author. All p values were two-sided, and results with $p < 0.05$ were considered significant.

Publication Output

Consider, first, the numbers and types of publications of the entire study cohort of 896 individuals, considered as if it were one group. A grand total of 1,580 classifiable articles was published in the tree target periods by members of the three clinical faculty groups (Table 5–4). Of these, 496 (31.4%) were reports on non-clinical research, and 1,084 (68.6%) fell into one of the seven categories of clinical research. In the aggregate, medicine and neurology had a considerably larger publication output than pediatrics, but the pediatricians published a larger proportion of their articles in clinical research. Approximately 90% of the clinical research reports dealt with studies in Categories 1 through 4 in all three departments: reports on management of disease (Category 2) predominated in the departments of medicine and pediatrics, while Basic POR (Category 1) articles led all other types in neurology. It is worth noting that reports on Basic and Applied POR (Categories 1 and 2) were twice as numerous as those dealing with the laboratory-based studies of Categories 3 and 4 (in vitro studies and models of disease, respectively) in all three departments, indicating the domi-

Table 5–4   Total Numbers of Research Articles Published by 896 Faculty Members in Three Clinical Departments in the Three Target Periods 1977–78, 1982–83, 1987–88[a]

	Total	Medicine	Pediatrics	Neurology
Total no. of publications	1,580	641	392	547
	(100)	(100)	(100)	(100)
Non-clinical research	496	203	92	201
	(31.4)	(31.7)	(24.5)	(36.7)
Clinical research (all seven categories)	1,084	438	300	346
	(68.6)	(68.3)	(75.5)	(63.3)
Cat. 1[b]	339	111	84	144
	(31.3)	(25.3)	(28.0)	(41.6)
Cat. 2[b]	355	158	109	88
	(32.7)	(36.1)	(36.3)	(25.4)
Cat. 3[b]	178	84	50	44
	(16.4)	(19.2)	(16.7)	(12.7)
Cat. 4[b]	109	55	25	29
	(10.0)	(12.6)	(8.3)	(8.4)
Cat. 5[b]	44	3	15	26
	(4.1)	(0.7)	(5.0)	(7.5)
Cat. 6[b]	36	17	9	10
	(3.3)	(3.9)	(3.0)	(2.9)
Cat. 7[b]	23	10	8	5
	(2.1)	(2.3)	(2.7)	(1.4)

[a]Total numbers and (in parentheses) percentages of the total number of publications.
[b]Totals in each category and (in parentheses) percentages of all clinical research publications.

nance of publications dealing with "bedside research" over "bench research" in this 10-year period.

The next two tables examine the differences among departments and trends that might have occurred over time. Table 5–5 shows a considerable increase in the total number of reports (all types over time in medicine and neurology, but not in pediatrics) and no consistent time trends for percentages of either non-clinical or clinical research articles except in neurology (where, for reasons that are not clear, non-clinical research reports significantly decreased and clinical research reports increased). Differences in the proportions of non-clinical and clinical articles among the three departments were small and not significant.

However, there were striking changes in the publications of the different categories of clinical research articles over time and among departments (Table 5–6). In all three departments, there were significant decreases in Basic POR (Category 1) articles, offset by increases in Applied POR (Category 2) articles in medicine and pediatrics but not in neurology. The proportions of clinical research articles published on strictly laboratory studies (Categories 3 and 4, summed) did not change over this 10-year period in any of the three departments. The far smaller numbers of research articles published in Categories 5, 6, and 7 (summed) increased somewhat in all three departments.

What is most striking about these data is the marked decline in attention to explorations of fundamental biologic questions in whole humans (Basic POR) in favor of an increasing emphasis on therapeutic trials (Applied POR). This waning attention to mechanistic questions and the increasing effort devoted to management-of-disease problems suggest a growing preference for certainty over uncertainty in clinical research. Publications dealing with laboratory-based research and animal models of human disease (Categories 3 and 4) did not increase systematically as Basic POR declined; this finding surprised me greatly because, as we shall see in Chapter 8, these non-patient categories of clinical research have been winning the lion's share of NIH grant support for clinical research over the last 10 years.

Changes in Faculty Ranks

This 3-D Survey also showed some interesting changes in the professional makeup of the three departments. On average, professors made up 36% of the total sample of 896 individuals, associate professors 31%, and assistant professors 33%; but, over time, there were decreasing proportions of full professors and increasing proportions of assistant professors in all three departments. For example, in medicine the proportion of full professors fell from 43 to 27% from 1977 to 1987, and that of assistant professors rose from 29 to 42%. The changes in neurology were even more striking: professors declined from 66 to 27% and assistant professors rose from 11 to 43%. This clearly reflects the growth in the size of all clinical departments through the hiring of younger staff members at lower ranks, which may explain in part the shift away from Basic POR over time in all departments that was shown in Table 5–6.

Table 5–5 Original Research Articles at Three Time Periods in Three Clinical Departments

	No. of Articles (and Percentages)						Percent of Clinical Research Articles in Each Category						
	All Types of Research		Non-Clinical Research		Clinical Research		1	2	3	4	5	6	7
Medicine													
1977–8	141	(100)	40	(28)	101	(72)	40	18	16	18	2	5	1
1982–3	153	(100)	52	(34)	101	(66)	31	39	18	9	1	3	0
1987–8	347	(100)	111	(32)	236	(68)	17	43	21	12	0	4	4
Total	641	(100)	203	(32)	438	(68)	b	b					
Pediatrics													
1977–8	102	(100)	17	(17)	85	(83)	41	26	6	6	4	6	1
1982–3	152	(100)	45	(30)	107	(70)	36	36	18	6	2	1	1
1987–8	138	(100)	30	(22)	108	(78)	9	44	16	13	9	3	6
Total	392	(100)	92	(24)	300	(77)	b	a					
Neurology													
1977–8	122	(100)	53	(43)	69	(57)	49	23	7	14	3	1	1
1982–3	161	(100)	78	(48)	83	(52)	51	17	11	11	1	7	2
1987–8	264	(100)	70	(27)	194	(74)	35	30	15	5	12	2	1
Total	547	(100)	201	(37)[b]	346	(63)[b]	a						
All Depts. (combined)													
1977–8	365	(100)	110	(30)	255	(70)	43	22	14	13	3	4	1
1982–3	466	(100)	175	(38)	291	(62)	38	32	16	8	1	3	1
1987–8	749	(100)	211	(28)	538	(72)	22	38	18	10	6	3	3
Total	1,580	(100)	496	(31)	1,084	(69)	b	b					

[a] $p < 0.01$ and [b] $p < 0.001$ in tests for trends over time.

Table 5–6   Original Articles on Clinical Research at Three Time Periods in Three Clinical Departments

	No. of Articles (and Percentages) in:								
	All Seven Categories		Category 1		Category 2		Categories 3 and 4		Categories 5–7
Medicine									
1977–8	101	(100)	41	(41)	18	(18)	34	(34)	8	(8)
1982–3	101	(100)	31	(31)	39	(39)	27	(27)	4	(4)
1987–8	236	(100)	39	(17)	101	(43)	78	(31)	18	(8)
Total	438	(100)	111	(25)[b]	158	(36)[b]	139	(32)	30	(7)
Pediatrics									
1977–8	85	(100)	35	(41)	22	(26)	19	(22)	9	(11)
1982–3	107	(100)	39	(36)	39	(36)	25	(23)	4	(4)
1987–8	108	(100)	10	(9)	48	(44)	31	(29)	19	(18)
Total	300	(100)	84	(28)[b]	109	(36)[b]	75	(25)	32	(11)
Neurology									
1977–8	69	(100)	34	(49)	16	(23)	15	(22)	4	(6)
1982–3	83	(100)	42	(51)	14	(17)	18	(22)	9	(11)
1987–8	194	(100)	68	(35)	58	(30)	40	(21)	28	(14)
Total	346	(100)	144	(45)[a]	88	(25)	73	(21)	41	(12)
All Depts. (combined)									
1977–8	255	(100)	110	(43)	56	(22)	68	(27)	21	(8)
1982–3	291	(100)	112	(39)	92	(32)	70	(24)	17	(6)
1987–8	538	(100)	117	(22)	207	(39)	149	(28)	65	(12)
Total	1,084	(100)	339	(31)[b]	355	(33)[b]	287	(27)	103	(10)[a]

[a] $p < 0.05$ and [b] $p < 0.0001$ in tests for trends over time.

Faculty Members as Authors

Of the 896 faculty members surveyed in the 3-D Survey, 453 (50.6%) published no research articles at all. A total of 443 others published at least one article on research: 158 (medicine), 131 (pediatrics), and 154 (neurology), out of approximately 300 faculty members sampled in each department (all time periods combined). The proportions of authors in *all* departments increased over time from 44 to 55% ($p < 0.01$) ("publish or perish"?), but this trend was significant only in medicine, where 46% of members published in 1977–78, rising to 62% in 1987–88. The number of publications per author also increased significantly over time in medicine (from a mean of 3.1 reports per author to 5.6) and neurology (2.5 to 4.6) ($p < 0.01$), but not in pediatrics (3.1 at both ends of the survey). The overall output of articles per author (all departments and all three time periods combined) rose from a mean of 2.9 to 4.6 ($p < 0.001$).

Table 5–7 shows that at least one article on non-clinical research was published by 36% of the 443 authors and on some form of clinical research by 86% of this group. There were no significant differences in the time trends of these ratios of non-clinical to clinical research authors among the three departments;

Table 5–7   3-D Survey of 443 Authors of Research Articles

	n	No. of Authors with at Least One Research Article In:				Percent of Clinical Research Authors with at Least One Research Article in Each of the Following Categories:			
		Non-Clinical Research		Clinical Research	Both	1	2	3	4
Medicine									
1977–8	46	19	⟨△⟩	40	13	45	30	28	28
1982–3	50	22	⟨△△⟩	41	13	39	54	27	12
1987–8	62	22	⟨△△△⟩	56	16	43	61	32	18
Totals	158	63	⟨△△△⟩	137	42		*b*		
% of total	100	40		87	27				
Pediatrics									
1977–8	36	8	⟨△△△⟩	34	6	50	50	24	9
1982–3	50	16	⟨△△△⟩	47	13	51	57	13	13
1987–8	45	15	⟨△△△⟩	37	7	19	73	35	16
Totals	131	39		118	26	*b*	*a*		
% of total	100	30		90	20				
Neurology									
1977–8	49	18	⟨△△△⟩	38	7	45	37	8	21
1982–3	48	16	⟨△△△⟩	39	7	54	31	10	8
1987–8	57	23	⟨△△△⟩	48	14	50	54	21	19
Totals	154	57	⟨△△△⟩	125	28				
% of total	100	37		81	18				
All Depts. (combined)									
1977–8	131	45	⟨△△△⟩	112	26	46	38	20	20
1982–3	148	54	⟨△△△⟩	127	33	48	48	17	11
1987–8	164	60	⟨△△△⟩	141	37	39	62	29	18
Totals	443	159	⟨△△△⟩	380	96		*b*		
% of total	100	36		86	22				

⟨△⟩ $p < 0.05$ in McNemar's tests of percentages right and left of this symbol.
⟨△△⟩ $p < 0.01$ in McNemar's tests of percentages right and left of this symbol.
⟨△△△⟩ $p < 0.001$ in McNemar's tests of percentages right and left of this symbol.
a$p < 0.05$ and *b*$p < 0.01$ in tests for trends over time.

but the large differences in the proportions of non-clinical to clinical research authors were significant in each time period in all three departments ($p < 0.05$ or less).

The 3-D Survey Summarized

The statistically significant (and unexpected) findings of this survey of the publication output of 896 faculty members in three major clinical departments, carried out at three time points over the period 1977–78, are as follows:

1. Only half of the faculty members published at least one research article of any type.
2. Clinical research articles outnumbered non-clinical research articles by 2 to 1, and purely laboratory-based studies numbered less than half of those dealing with POR (Table 5–4).
3. There were no time trends in the ratios of non-clinical to clinical research articles in medicine or pediatrics, but in neurology there was a significant increase in clinical research publications and a significant decrease in non-clinical research publications (Table 5–5).
4. The percentages of Basic POR articles (Category 1) decreased significantly in all three departments over time, and Applied POR articles (Category 2) increased significantly in medicine and pediatrics (Table 5–6).
5. The proportion of authors of clinical research articles in all departments at all three time points exceeded the proportion of authors of non-clinical research articles by more than 2 to 1 ($p < 0.05$ or less) (Table 5–7).
6. Significant increases over time were found in Category 2 (Applied POR) authors in medicine and pediatrics, and a significant decrease was found in Category 1 (Basic POR) authors only in pediatrics (Table 5–7).
7. There were no time trends in the number of authors reporting laboratory-based studies (Categories 3 and 4) in any of the three departments (Table 5–7).

The 3-D Survey demonstrates that large numbers of full-time members of major clinical departments are not engaged in any sort of original research; this reflects the continued growth in the size of clinical faculties for sake of income generation rather than for research. Further, the survey reveals that Basic POR activity over the period 1977–87 was replaced by Applied POR (but not by bench research, Categories 3 and 4), which reflects a growing avoidance of risk-taking and increasing reliance on certainty in clinical research among major clinical faculties of U.S. medical schools. (Later chapters will support these impressions.)

(Some observers have argued that Category 4—animal models of human disease—ought not to be classified as clinical research, although I disagree on this point; see Chapter 4. However, giving the benefit of doubt to that argument, a second test was performed. All Category 4 authors were shifted into the non-clinical research columns of Table 5–7; the differences in the proportions of non-clinical and clinical research authors noted in item 5 above remained significant in seven of nine analyses, but not for medicine and neurology in 1977–78.)

Not shown in Tables 5–4 to 5–7 was the unsurprising finding that, in all three departments at all three time periods, the number of faculty members publishing at least one research article was largest in those institutions ranked as most research-intensive, coupled with the smallest number of non-publishing faculty members. For example, the ratio of authors to non-authors in the top third of the intensity rank order was 1.7 to 1, and in the bottom third it was 1 to 0.65.

A SURVEY OF RESEARCH PRODUCTIVITY AT THE
NIH CLINICAL CENTER

The Clinical Center at NIH was set up in 1953 to complement the existing laboratory facilities of the eight Institutes established at that time, with the express purpose of making it possible to conduct POR in ways not readily available to researchers at U.S. medical schools. As will be shown in Chapter 6, the Clinical Center, with its 500 beds and out-patient facilities, contains in one building almost as many beds for research purposes as exist throughout the rest of the country.

The clinician-scientists engaged in research at the Clinical Center have two main advantages over those in U.S. medical schools. First, supported as they are by internal funding, they do not compete with their peers nationwide for grant monies. Second, and even more important, they are not distracted from their research by teaching or by providing clinical service to the general public, as are MD-researchers in U.S. medical schools. However, they labor under one disadvantage: their research efforts are not reviewed internally with the same rigor that typifies the peer reviews of competitive grants and of clinical research centers outside Bethesda, Maryland.

In view of these differences from the condition of clinicians whose research productivity was measured in the 3-D Survey, I felt it would be illuminating to study the publication output of a highly selected group of Clinical Center physician-scientists in order to demonstrate the level and type of research productivity that can be attained in the absence of the time- and fiscal constraints that exist in U.S. medical schools.

Personal interviews were arranged in early 1989 with each of the clinical directors of the 12 Institutes that were then utilizing the facilities of the NIH Clinical Center. Each of them was asked to name the three MDs (or MD-PhDs) who made the *largest and best* use of the in- or out-patient facilities assigned to that Institute. Confidentiality was promised and fully observed. I then performed the same type of publication review described in the 3-D Survey; the target year was 1988, and the Medline search and analysis of abstracts of original research articles was completed by late 1989. The same exclusions pertained in this CC Survey: case reports, hospital record reviews, literature reviews, book chapters, and preliminary publications reported only as abstracts.

Thirty-six physician-scientists had been named by the 12 clinical directors: three had no research publications recorded in the Medline system in 1988. For the remaining 33 scientists, I found 220 research articles that were classifiable, a mean publication rate of 6.7 articles per author in this highly selected sample of researchers (in contrast to 4.6 in the strictly randomized 3-D Survey).

Looking at the data first in terms of the number of physician-scientists who published at least one article in particular categories of research, we find the following (Table 5–8):

Table 5–8 Number of Authors Publishing at Least One Article in:

	CC Survey (1988)		3-D Survey (1987–88) (Three Departments Combined)	
	No.	% of Total	No.	% of Total
Total no. of authors	33	100	164	100
Non-clinical research	18	55	60	37
Clinical research (all categories)	31	94	141	86
Category 1	22	67	55	34
Category 2	19	58	87	53
Category 3	11	33	41	25
Category 4	15	45	25	15
Categories 5–7	8	24	27	19

What is strikingly different in the research preferences of the Clinical Center scientists compared to those in U.S. medical schools is the larger percentage of Clinical Center authors reporting on Basic POR and, at the same time, on non-clinical research.

Table 5–9 presents an analysis of the 220 research articles of the 33 physician-scientists and their classification into one of the seven categories of clinical research. In this optimal environment for biomedical research, 76% of the research publications dealt with some form of clinical research, and the largest percentage of this group dealt with Basic POR (Category 1). Reports on Applied POR (management of disease, Category 2), which included therapeutic trials of all sorts, did *not* outnumber those in Category 1, as they did in 1987–88 in the 3-D Survey. However, the aggregate of the laboratory studies in Categories 3

Table 5–9 Original Articles on Biomedical Research Published in 1988 by 33 Selected Physician-Scientists of the 12 National Institutes of Health on Studies Performed at the NIH Clinical Center

	Total[a]	Non-Clin.	Clin.	Seven Categories of Clinical Research						
				1	2	3	4	5	6	7
No. of articles	220	52	168	62	33	29	30	5	8	1
Percent of all research articles	100	23.6	76.4	28	15	13	14	2	4	—
Percent of clinical research articles			100	37	20	17	18	3	5	—

[a]Exclusive of case reports, hospital record reviews, abstracts, reviews, and book chapters.

and 4 (in vitro studies and animal models) was considerably larger (35% of clinical research articles) than that found in the 3-D Survey (26%). The tally for Categories 1 through 4 was 92% for the Clinical Center researchers, as it was in the 3-D Survey (Table 5–7), indicating for both study cohorts the small amount of research effort focused on field trials, developmental research, and outcomes research.

THE REAL WORLD AND THE IVORY TOWER

The 3-D and CC Surveys compare the various kinds of biomedical research undertaken recently in U.S. medical schools with those in the protected research conditions of the NIH Clinical Center—the real world versus the ivory tower. Constrained seriously and increasingly by demands on their time for activities other than research, physician-scientists in medical schools have been turning away from Basic POR to protocols dealing with the management of disease (Applied POR). In contrast, the prominence of Basic POR in the research of physician-scientists in the Clinical Center illustrates what can be accomplished in the absence of the constraints that burden physician-scientists in the real world.

If the research activities of U.S. physician-scientists in the future can be divined from the distribution pattern of traditional research project grants (RO1 grants) in recent years, current trends away from Basic POR will increasingly demonstrate the choice of scientists in the real world to concentrate on animal models of human disease (Category 4) and in vitro studies of materials of human origin (Category 3), both of which are less time-intensive research activities than is POR. These indications will be examined in the next two chapters, which deal with the NIH and its grants system.

SUMMARY AND CONCLUSIONS

The size of the pool of biomedical researchers in the United States today is not easily measured because MDs (in particular) have many responsibilities other than research that compete for their time. The best estimate of the number of MD and PhD researchers lies between 12,000 and 32,000, of whom about half are MDs.

Departments of medicine in U.S. medical schools are considered to be major sites of biomedical research, yet a recent survey (Gentile, 1987) showed that only one-third of their full-time staffs spent as much as 20% of their time in research, had outside funding for and space allocated to their research, and produced one or more research papers in 2 years.

That 1987 descriptive survey did not examine the nature of the research performed by these clinical investigators (reductionist, integrative, or non-clinical), so a special study was designed to clarify this point. A random sample of MD and PhD faculty members of three clinical departments (medicine, pediatrics, and neurology) was selected at three time periods between 1977 and 1987. The abstracts of all their research articles were read, and were assigned to one of the seven categories of clinical research or to the category of non-clinical research. Half of the sample population of 900 full-time faculty members published no research articles at all; the other half reported about 1,600 research reports in the three target periods combined. Three times as many authors described some form of clinical research compared to non-clinical research, and about 40% published at least one article on Basic POR. However, over the 10-year period, the number of Basic POR authors declined precipitously in pediatrics, and in medicine the number of Applied POR authors doubled. In all three departments, there were significant downward trends over time in the number of publications in Basic POR, and increases in Applied POR in medicine and pediatrics.

The reasons for these trends in the type of clinical research performed in major clinical departments of U.S. medical schools—away from time-intensive, risk-taking mechanistic studies of human biology toward the performance of management-of-disease studies that are less time-intensive and far more certain in outcome—reflect the radical change in mores in these schools that have followed the shrinkage in funding for young investigators, the pressure on them to publish or perish, the time constraints created by demands on them for income generation through medical services to patients, and the allure of new technologies of bench research that are more likely to win grant support, promotions, and tenure. A contrasting study of research publications at the NIH Clinical Center, where physician-scientists are not burdened by the time constraints of teaching or income generation or medical service to the general public, confirmed these conclusions.

APPENDIX: METHODOLOGY OF THE 3-D SURVEY

Using the AAMC Faculty Roster System, a random selection was made of 100 names in 1977, 1982, and 1987 in each of the three departments to yield nine sets of 100 names each. The survey was limited to active full-time faculty members with MD or MD-PhD degrees holding the rank of professor, associate professor, or assistant professor. The Faculty Roster yielded all this (and much other) information on the total number of faculty members in these clinical departments (the "universe"), from which the random samples were selected (Table 5–10).

Reports for which authors' abstracts were on record in the NML's Medline system were called up for review in three 2-year publication periods: 1977 and 1978, 1982 and 1983, and 1987 and 1988. (The survey could not be carried out at earlier time periods, because the Medline system furnished a complete recall of abstracts written in English only after 1976.) After verifying the correctness of all name identifications in terms of initials, institutions, and research interests, as indicated by publication titles and abstracts, 4 names out of 900 were discarded because of confusing or incomplete information. Thus, the nine study

Table 5–10   Numbers of Medically Trained Full-Time Faculty Members with Ranks of Professor, Associate Professor, and Assistant Professor in Three Clinical Departments in All U.S. Medical Schools

	1977	1982	1987
Medicine			
Total (universe)	8,723	10,196	10,778
MDs	8,103	9,405	9,934
MD-PhDs	620	791	844
% MD-PhDs	7.1	7.8	7.8
Study cohort*a*	100	99	100
Pediatrics			
Total (universe)	3,643	4,188	4,463
MDs	3,458	3,936	4,197
MD-PhDs	185	252	266
% MD-PhDs	5.1	6.0	6.0
Study cohort*a*	99	99	99
Neurology			
Total (universe)	1,001	1,161	1,203
MDs	906	1,033	1,055
MD-PhDs	95	128	146
% MD-PhDs	9.4	11.0	12.1
Study cohort*a*	100	100	100

*a*Number of faculty members randomly selected from the universe for the 3-D Survey.

Source: AAMC Faculty Roster System (Drs. Paul Jolly and Brooke Whiting, personal communication).

samples with a total of 896 names represented selections of 1% of the total U.S. faculties of medicine, 2.4% (pediatrics), and 8.9% (neurology). MD-PhDs made up some 7% of the sample (compared to an average of 8.6% in the three universes), with (on average) 8.8% in neurology, 6.7% in medicine, and 5.1% in pediatrics; there were no apparent time trends in these percentages.

Having correctly identified each faculty member, I read the titles and abstracts of all publications during the target years of the 896 faculty members selected as described and coded each report into one of eight possible groups: 1 through 7 for the seven categories of clinical research, and a separate one for non-clinical research (all as defined in Chapter 4). Counts were not made of reports lacking abstracts, or of case reports, hospital record reviews, reviews of the scientific literature, or book chapters, since I had chosen (Chapter 3) not to regard these types of publications as reSEARCH; these non-tallied publications were always easily identifiable. I then summed all counts for each individual and entered these counts into a separate database for further calculations.

6

The National Institutes of Health and National Health Expenditures

As U.S. campuses go, that of the National Institutes of Health (NIH) is by no means the largest—in acreage or in numbers of buildings, faculty, and students (NIH Almanac, NIH Pub. No. 88-5). But as a center for biomedical science it is certainly the largest in the world, and arguably the most prestigious.

Located in Bethesda, Maryland, some 8 miles northwest of the capital on rich suburban land privately owned until 1935, the 40 (mostly) red brick buildings of the NIH sit on some 306 acres of carefully landscaped ground and provide their 10,000 personnel with some 5.2 million square feet of laboratory, office, and hospital space (or 120 acres of floor area). In 1988 the NIH community consisted of about 1,600 MDs, 2,000 PhDs, 170 with other doctoral degrees, and more than 6,000 civil service employees. It boasts its own underground station, which allows travelers to reach the center of the District of Columbia in about 20 minutes and the National Airport in 35 minutes. There are 12 miles of roadways on the campus and some 8,800 parking spaces, as well as jitney buses that move at regular intervals from building to building and from the center of the campus to the National Library of Medicine, an adjoining component of the NIH that is a treasure in its own right. The administrative staff has grown so large that the overflow has been moved to a satellite office building 2 miles away.

The National Institutes are now 13 in number, each with its own director and with deputy directors who oversee their separate intramural and extramural activities. In addition, there are four major divisions (Research Grants, Research Resources, Research Services, and Computer Research), as well as the National Library of Medicine and three Centers (Fogarty International, Nursing Research, and the Warren Magnuson Clinical Center). The campus also houses the Food and Drug Administration's Center for Biologics Evaluation and two components of the Alcohol, Drug Abuse, and Mental Health Administration (ADAMHA), namely, the National Institute of Alcohol Abuse and Alcoholism and the National Institute of Mental Health.

The mission of the NIH is described as follows (IOM Committee Report, 1988a): "to improve the health of the nation by increasing the understanding of processes underlying human health, disability, and disease, advancing knowledge concerning the health effects of interaction between man and the environment, and developing and improving methods of preventing, detecting, diagnosing, and treating disease." This cumbersome but global mandate directs the NIH to investigate all aspects of human biology for the sake of guarding and improving the nation's health. Each step in the history of the NIH has been taken with the sanction of Congress.

ONE HUNDRED YEARS OF GROWTH AND DEVELOPMENT

In 1988 the NIH celebrated its 100th anniversary with a year-long gala devoted to its spectacular record of achievements. Beginning as a one-room laboratory in the Marine Hospital on Staten Island, New York, the Hygiene Laboratory was moved to Washington, D.C., in 1891 and charged with the investigation of communicable diseases under the aegis of the Surgeon General of the Public Health Service. With a broadened mandate, the laboratory became involved in nutritional deficiency disorders, then venereal diseases, and later drug addiction. In 1930 its name was changed to the National Institute of Health. Two new buildings were constructed in downtown Washington, D.C., and training fellowships were initiated. In 1935 the first of several gifts of land in Bethesda, Maryland, was made by Mr. and Mrs. Luke I. Wilson—45 acres at first, and 92 acres in all by 1942; this is now the nucleus of the NIH campus. The National Cancer Institute was set up as an independent unit by Congress in 1937 and was joined to the NIH by legislation in 1944.

During World War II, a wide range of scientific studies was carried out by scientists throughout the United States under a contract with the National Research Council's Office of Scientific Research and Development (OSRD), headed by Vannevar Bush. With the end of the war in sight, Thomas Parran, Surgeon General of the Public Health Service, set up a panel of experts headed by W.W. Palmer of Columbia University's College of Physicians and Surgeons to consider the post-war disposition of the many OSRD contracts. Palmer's committee recommended the formation of a new agency to manage these contracts; in due course, an Office of Research Grants was established in 1946 under Rolla E. Dyer, the director of the NIH. This new office was administered by C.J. Van Slyke and given an additional charge: to establish a program of extramural research grants and fellowship awards. Van Slyke was responsible for setting up a system of extramural study sections for review of grant applications, a peer review process that is still in place today and hailed as one of the great achievements of the NIH. It was an innovation of major importance for ensuring healthy relationships between government and the academic world.

With the formation by Congress of the National Heart Institute and the National Institute for Dental Research in 1948, the name of the NIH was changed from Institute to Institutes, and over the next 42 years the number of separate Institutes grew from 3 to 13. The Clinical Center of the NIH was opened in

1955, with some 500 beds and all the support services that a general hospital requires. However, it was set up only to serve the research interests of the various Institutes, and it remains a unique resource for studies in human beings to which patients are admitted strictly by invitation of the clinical staffs of the various Institutes.

When the Soviets launched Sputnik in 1957, the U.S. Congress responded with an unprecedented surge of appropriations for science. Deftly guided by Senators Lester Hill and Warren Magnuson, Congressman John Fogarty, Mrs. Mary Lasker, NIH director James A. Shannon, and their many friends outside Congress, ever-increasing appeals to Congress for funds for biomedical research were extraordinarily successful. At the same time, funds were also allocated for construction of new hospitals and medical schools, experimental field stations, and other research resources. Senator Paul Douglas (D., Ill.), speaking of Senator Hill (D., Ala.), said that he "touches the rock of public credit and abundant streams rush forth, so that the NIH have more money running out of their ears, money they do not always know what to do with" (quoted in Strickland, 1972). That post-Sputnik decade is often referred to as the golden era of biomedical research in the United States. The $500,000 appropriation to the NIH in 1938 doubled by 1943 and continued to double 14 times, reaching a total of $8 billion in 1989.

Lewis Thomas (1981) has called the NIH the "most brilliant social invention of the twentieth century." Indeed, the influence of the NIH has been felt in almost every aspect of American life—social, technological, economic, academic, and industrial (as well as medical). It has been studied, criticized, and admired throughout the world. Like all large enterprises, it has taken on a life of its own. Starting as an organization devoted with great modesty to the service of scientists throughout the United States, it has grown into an empire that has become the main source of nourishment of biomedical science in the United States, with an ever-larger treasury of funds but also an increasing number of bureaucratic controls.

Although the NIH is centrally administered by a director and a deputy director, the 13 individual Institutes, each named for a disease of major interest, are almost autonomous, especially in their relationships with congressional funding committees. The several Institutes are tied to the central NIH director's office on matters of common interest through the oversight of the Deputy Director for Intramural Research and the Deputy Director for Extramural Research and Training. The latter director, in turn, is served by some nine associate directors in charge of specific programs and activities of general NIH interest, and they, in turn, by at least 20 division directors. The complexity of this administrative structure is justified by the size of its $8 billion budget, by the need to account to Congress for its annual appropriations, and by a complex process of establishing annual budgets (a 2-year process that moves in several steps from NIH to Congress and to the Office of Management and Budget of the President's Office).

The NIH director answers to the Secretary of the Department of Health and Human Services (DHHS) through an Assistant Secretary for Health. The directors of the 13 Institutes and other senior officials of the NIH are appointed by the Secretary of DHHS, except for the director of the National Cancer Institute, whose appointment, like that of the NIH director, is made by the president and confirmed by Congress.

THE 13 INSTITUTES

In 1948, when construction of the Clinical Center was begun, the NIH consisted of only three Institutes: Cancer, Heart, and Dental Research. By 1953, when the first patient was admitted to the Clinical Center, five more Institutes had been formed: Microbiology, Experimental Biology and Medicine, Mental Health, Neurological Diseases and Blindness, and Arthritis and Metabolic Diseases. There has been a series of mergers, separations, and re-namings since 1953. By 1990 there were 12 Institutes on the NIH campus and one (Environmental Health Sciences) located in Research Triangle Park, North Carolina (Table 6–1). The National Institute of Mental Health (NIMH), originally in NIH, was shifted to the jurisdiction of another DHHS bureau, ADAMHA, in 1967; NIMH maintains its clinical activities and a large part of its laboratory work on the NIH campus.

Each of the Institutes is organized under a director, who oversees the activities of a scientific director and a clinical director. Each Institute's budget is separately negotiated with Congress (funds appropriated to the individual Insti-

Table 6–1   The 13 Institutes of the NIH in 1990[a]

Date	Full Name	Abbreviation
1937	National Cancer Institute	NCI
1948	National Heart, Lung, and Blood Institute	NHLBI
1948	National Institute of Dental Research	NIDR
1950	National Institute of Diabetes and Digestive and Kidney Diseases	NIADDK
1950	National Institute of Neurological Disorders and Stroke	NINDS
1955	National Institute of Allergy and Infectious Diseases	NIAID
1962	National Institute of General Medical Sciences	NIGMS
1962	National Institute of Child Health and Human Development	NICHD
1968	National Eye Institute	NEI
1969	National Institute of Environmental Health Sciences	NIEHS
1974	National Institute on Aging	NIA
1985	National Institute of Arthritis and Musculoskeletal and Skin Diseases	NIAMS
1988	National Institute of Deafness and Other Communication Disorders	NIDCD

[a]Listed in order of their authorization by Congress.

tutes cannot be interchanged). Each Institute director meets at least three times each year with an Advisory Council of outsiders whose appointments are approved by the president; these councils set policy for their individual Institutes and are the final arbiters on all extramural awards. Each scientific director also meets at least three times each year with a Board of Scientific Counselors of outside scientists (Cancer has four such boards); the clinical directors answer to their scientific directors and seek outsiders' opinions and counsel only rarely, and then on an ad hoc basis.

Each of the Institutes carries out selective recruitment of young investigators, both PhDs and MDs: these research associates and clinical associates remain in training at the NIH for about 3 years before moving elsewhere. The intramural activities of the several Institutes are organized according to the preferences of the individual directors; the degree of collegiality among the staff members of a given Institute varies greatly, as do the relationships between the clinical and laboratory scientists of any one Institute. While in principle the intramural bench and bedside staffs have the opportunity to engage in productive collaborative research, this design is frequently thwarted by the size of the institution, by the separateness of the Institutes from each other, by the location of laboratories at considerable distances from each other, by the lack of communal facilities that might promote closer interpersonal relationships, and by a high degree of competitiveness among the staffs at all levels. While these barriers can be and have been overcome by strong leadership, this has been the exception, not the rule.

The extramural activities of each Institute account for the expenditure of most of their annual appropriation. They are administered by a staff that is separate from the intramural staff and that works closely with scientists outside the NIH in oversight of specialized centers, program projects, training grants and fellowship awards, and competitive research grants. The extramural staffs themselves are not engaged in laboratory or clinical research, but act chiefly as liaison with outside scientists in carrying out the missions of their individual Institutes.

The 13 Institutes vary greatly in the sizes of their budgets, number of professional personnel, and space allocations for laboratories and clinical facilities. Table 6–2 demonstrates some of these differences among the 11 Institutes on the NIH campus in 1977–87. Intramural costs in 1987 varied from 0.1 to 27.7% of their annual obligations, and annual obligations varied from $59 to $705 million. NCI (Cancer) had the largest appropriation and, except for NIDR and NIEHS, spent the largest amount of its appropriation on intramural activities. NIGMS (General Medical Sciences) has no intramural laboratory or clinical program and spends its appropriation almost entirely on grants and training programs.

Not shown on Table 6–2 are the numbers of permanent full-time personnel in the several Institutes. In 1988 they ranged from 29 to 321 for those in the offices of the (then) 11 Institute directors, and from 27 to 1,171 for those engaged in intramural research. There was a total complement of 10,765 full-time personnel in the entire NIH, exclusive of some 3,900 staff fellows and visiting scientists.

Table 6–2 Intramural and Extramural Obligations of the NIH (in Millions of Dollars)

Total NIH Obligations	1977	1982	1987
Current dollars	2,582	3,643	6,175
Constant 1977 dollars	2,582	2,362	3,101
% intramural	9.6	12.4	10.8

Intramural Expenditures of 11 Institutes[a] (in Millions of 1977 Dollars and as a Percentage of Total Institute Obligations)	1977	1982	1987
NCI	$815	639	705
	12.6%	17.2%	17.5%
NHLBI	396	363	467
	8.2	8.6	6.8
NIAID	140	153	274
	19.8	18.2	13.2
NICHD	145	146	184
	10.7	11.5	11.2
NINCDS	155	172	246
	15.0	14.8	11.2
NIADDK	219	239	257
	14.1	12.9	11.3
NEI	64	84	108
	11.0	9.7	8.6
NIA	30	53	89
	20.4	7.6	3.0
NIDR	55	47	59
	19.2	20.0	20.6
NIEHS	51	69	105
	26.4	27.4	27.7
NIGMS	205	220	287
	0.2	0.2	0.1

[a]NIMH is not listed here; it is a component of ADAMHA (not NIH); the newest Institutes (NIAMS and NIDCD) were not set up until 1985 and 1988, respectively.

Source: *IOM Committee Report: A Healthy NIH Intramural Program* (1988a), Table 1–1.

THE WARREN MAGNUSON CLINICAL CENTER

In 1987, the Clinical Center had 495 beds assigned to 12 Institutes on the basis of need and precedence. In many respects, the Clinical Center operated as if it were 12 separate research hospitals, but certain administrative features tied these 12 units together. The Clinical Center's director and his supporting staff are responsible for the 2- to 3-year appointments of the approximately 125 medical staff fellows selected by the individual Institutes, for medical student fellowships in the summer months, for a program that brings normal volunteers into research studies at the Clinical Center, and for review of the safety and efficacy of all research projects undertaken throughout the Center by all the Institutes. In addition, the Clinical Center's director oversees the several facilities that service the general medical needs of the entire Center, such as pharmacy, radiology, blood bank, critical care unit, physical therapy, and outpatient research facilities.

The bed allocations to the 12 user Institutes in 1987 are shown in Table 6–3. (NIMH and NIAAA are included in Table 6–3 as users, although they are administratively attached to ADAMHA, not to NIH.) Allocations varied from 117 beds in the NCI to 4 beds in the NIDR. This table also sets out the rank

Table 6–3 Size Relationships and FY1987 Obligations for Intramural Research of the 12 Institutes Using the Clinical Center[a]

All 12 Institutes	Research Personnel[b]		Total Intramural Research Obligations
	No. of FTEs	Personnel Costs	
Totals	4,972	$228,404,000	$665,311,000
% of total		34.3%	100%

Individual Institutes	Allocated Beds			Percent of Total Intramural Obligations[f]					
				Research FTE's		Personnel Costs		Total Research Costs	
	No.	%	Rank Order	%	Rank Order	%	Rank Order	%	Rank Order
NCI	117	24	1	35.8	1	38.4	1	40.3	1
NHLBI	89	18	2	9.2	5	8.2	5	10.5	3
NIMH[c]	57	12	3						
NIAID	50	10	4	12.1	2	10.9	2	11.9	2
NICHD	44	9	5	6.0	6	6.5	6	6.7	6
NINCDS	43	9	6	11.2	3	10.3	4	9.0	5
NIADDK	40	8	7	10.0	4	10.8	3	9.5	4
NIAMS[d]	16	3	8	0.9	10	0.9	10	1.1	10
NEI	12	2	9	3.2	9	3.2	9	3.1	9
NIAAA[c]	10	2	10						
NIA	6	1	11	5.7	8	5.3	8	3.8	8
NIDR	4	1	12	6.0	7	5.4	7	4.0	7
Clin. Cnt.[e]	7	1							
Totals	495	100		100.1		99.9		99.9	

[a]Data furnished by the NIH Division of Financial Management, December 1988 (Warren Bock).

[b]MDs, PhDs, technicians, and secretaries (research personnel only).

[c]Components of ADAMHA (not NIH).

[d]Activated in 1985.

[e]The critical care unit of the Clinical Center.

[f]After deduction of expenditures of NIEHS and NIGMS, which do not utilize the Clinical Center.

orders of the 12 Institutes in terms of their research personnel, personnel costs, and total research costs. Although the NCI was first in all rankings, the correlation between bed allocations and the three other parameters was far from tight. However, the rankings of the three measures of total intramural obligations correlated rather well with each other from Institute to Institute, which is not surprising since personnel costs make up such a large part of total research costs (34.3%).

NIH AND THE NATIONAL HEALTH BUDGET

The money spent on the nation's health is said to be the largest single item in the U.S. economy: $500 billion in 1987, or 11% of the GNP (Fuchs, 1990). In constant dollars, total health costs rose 34% from 1980 to 1989 (an annual growth rate of 6.1%), which is three times greater than that for expenditures for total health research and development (*NIH Data Book*, 1990).

To orient ourselves in regard to the part played by the NIH in the total U.S. expenditure for health research and development (R&D), we note that expenditures for total health R&D in 1989 were 3.7% of the total health costs in the United States and that the NIH budget was 34% of total health R&D. In other words, the NIH budget was 1.2% of total health costs. Figure 6–1 shows the major sources of the national support for health R&D. While all sources have

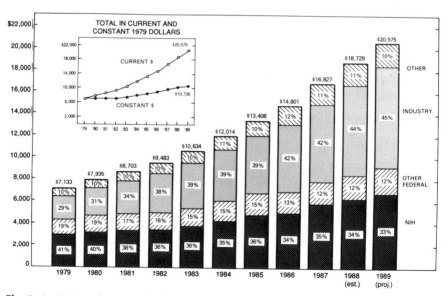

Fig. 6–1 National support for health R&D by source, 1979–89 (dollars in millions). (*NIH Data Book*, 1989, Fig. 2.1)

increased in current dollars as well as in constant dollars, the proportion spent by the NIH has decreased from 41% in 1979 to 33% in 1988, and "other federal" expenditures have fallen from 19 to 12%. In contrast, the industry source has grown from 29 to 45%. In evaluating these changes, we must recognize that for industry (primarily the pharmaceutical and biotechnology industries), D monies far exceed R monies. This is the reverse of the NIH situation, where D is minor, R major.

An explanation of the "other federal" category, which now makes up 12% of national health R&D dollars, is in order. "Other federal" signifies the non-NIH dollars spent by DHSS, plus the dollars spent by other federal agencies on health R&D. Table 6–4 makes the point that federal agencies other than DHHS spend 7.7% of the total commitment of the nation to health R&D, in contrast to NIH's 35%.

Ginzberg and Dutka (1989) refer to "biomedical R&D" rather than "health R&D" (the NIH usage); their analyses of the trends in national expenditures for biomedical R&D from 1940 to 1987 are shown in Figs. 6–2 and 6–3. The striking increase in constant dollars over this 47-year period, and especially in the last 5 years (Fig. 6–2), has been due in large part to increased expenditures by

Table 6–4 National Support for Health R&D, 1989

		Dollars (in Millions)	Percent of Total
DHHS Support for NIH alone		5,851.0	34.8
Other Federal Support		1,976.0	11.7
Other DHHS (non-NIH)		(687.0)	(4.1)
Other federal agencies		(1,289.0)	(7.7)
Agriculture	99.3		
Defense	407.1		
Energy	177.1		
Environmental Protection	49.3		
AID	33.7		
Aeronautics & Space	131.6		
NSF	89.9		
Veterans	209.5		
Other	91.5		
Industry Support		7,130.0	42.4
All Other Support		1,831.4	11.1
State & local govts.	1,146.0		(6.8)
Nonprofit	725.0		(4.3)
Total		16,649.0	100.0

Source: *NIH Data Book* (1989), Tables 2 and 4.

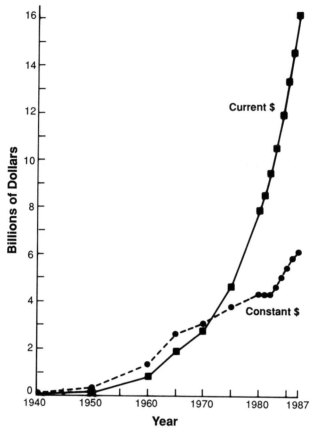

Fig. 6–2 National funds for biomedical R&D, 1940–87 (current and constant 1940 dollars, in billions). (Ginzberg and Dutka, 1989, Fig. 2.1; based on the *NIH Data Book,* 1988)

industry (Fig. 6–3). Consequently the proportion of total biomedical R&D dollars contributed by the federal government has dropped and that from private philanthropy has leveled off.

   Those who analyze the impacts of these events stress that the only flexibility in the national budget lies in the reduction of federal expenditures for defense. Table 6–5a shows that, if the defense budget remains at 22% of the federal budget (as was projected for 1991), discretionary spending can make up no more than 16% of a budget manipulated by Congress to meet all its many priorities, only one of which is biomedical research. Recent events in Eastern Europe raised the hope that the U.S. defense budget could be reduced, but this expectation grew dim when the Persian Gulf crisis occurred. The many programs that compete for attention by the congressional committees that control the annual appropriation to the NIH are shown in Table 6–5b. Despite this competition for fund-

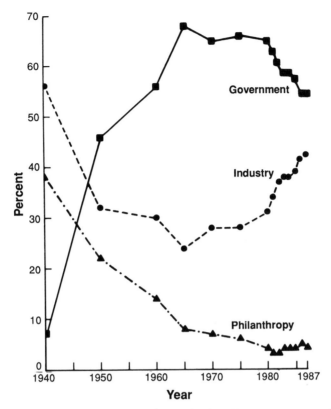

Fig. 6–3 Sources of national funds for biomedical R&D as percentages of the total, 1940–87. (Ginzberg and Dutka, 1989, Fig. 2.2; based on the *NIH Data Book*, 1988)

ing, in 1991 the NIH appropriation amounted to 3.8% of non-defense discretionary spending; this percentage has been growing steadily since 1981, at an annual rate of 6.7%.

Thus, the amount of money devoted to health R&D in the United States has risen constantly, but not nearly so rapidly as the nation's total health costs. Although the proportion of total health R&D costs derived from the NIH has decreased constantly over the last 10 years compared to that of industry, the annual appropriation to NIH by Congress has consistently increased in constant dollars, but also as a percentage of non-defense discretionary spending. We have already noted the confusion that can arise when R&D figures are presented as a single number (how much is R, how much D?) and when sources of all national funds for biomedical R&D are presented as proportions rather than as totals (as exemplified by Fig. 6–3). In fact, the dollars appropriated by Congress to NIH after 1982 have increased strikingly. Figure 6–4 shows these increases plotted in terms of constant dollars.

Table 6–5a Allocation of the Federal Budget by Major Spending Categories

Fiscal Year	Total Federal Operating Budget (Current $) (Billions)	National Defense	Entitlements and Other Mandatory Spending	Net Interest on the Debt	Non-defense Discretionary Spending	NIH Appropriation (Current $) (Millions)
1981	678	23%	41%	10%	25%	3,333
1984	852	27	41	13	19	4,258
1988	1064	27	42	14	17	6,291
1991	1363	22	47	14	16	8,307

Source: Congressional Budget Office (personal communication, Paul N. Van de Water, December 1990).

Table 6–5b Some Programs Funded in the Labor/HHS/Education Appropriations Bill in Addition to NIH

Aid to Families with Dependent Children	AIDS Treatment, Prevention Efforts
Centers for Disease Control	Childhood Immunization Programs
Community and Migrant Health Care Centers	Education Programs
Health Care for the Homeless	Heating Assistance for Low Income Households
Infant Mortality Initiatives	Maternal and Child Health Block Grants
National Council on the Handicapped	Nurse Training
Occupational Safety and Health Administration	Primary Care Physician Training

Source: AFCR Newsletter, 1989; 1(2), Table 3.

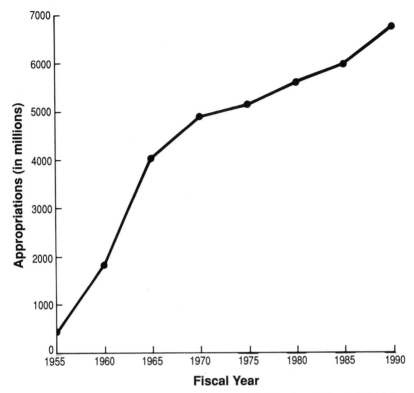

Fig. 6–4 Total NIH appropriations (constant 1988 dollars, in millions). (*IOM Report on Research Funding: A Strategy to Restore Balance,* 1990, Table A–2, abbreviated)

TRENDS IN NIH SPENDING

Over the years, there have been some important trends in the extramural spending of NIH, which makes up about 89% of the total NIH appropriation. These trends are shown in Fig. 6–5. Over the period 1972–86, training funds decreased steadily from 13 to 5%, and traditional research projects increased from 44 to 66%. R&D contracts grew from 18 to 23% in 1975 but declined thereafter to 10%, while the monies for centers and other targeted research remained constant at about 20%. Most observers applaud the growth in funding of traditional research projects, for these (as we will discuss later) are the main source of support for individual biomedical scientists.

The AAMC describes this trend somewhat differently. Table 6–6 shows the balance between investigator-initiated and nationally targeted research from 1960 to 1988. In the Nixon era, targeted research reached its maximum in 1975 at 41% of extramural awards, then fell below 30% after 1982. Investigator-initiated research was highest in 1960 (at 86% of all awards); then, as targeted research increased in the 1970s, it fell to its lowest level (59%); since 1975 it has risen again to 75% of all awards.

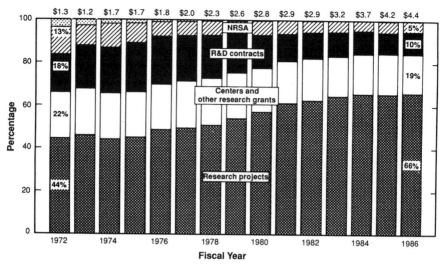

Fig. 6–5 Allocation of NIH extramural awards by activity, FY1972–86 (in percentages of total amounts awarded, with current dollars in billions). (Wyngaarden, 1987, Fig. 3. These data have been updated for FY1989 as follows: NRSA 4%, R&D contracts 11%, Centers 17%, and Research Projects 67%. From *DRG Extramural Trends, FY1980–89*, p. 6)

Table 6–6 Distribution of NIH Obligations (in Millions of Current Dollars)

Fiscal Year	Total Research	Investigator-Initiated Research		Nationally Targeted Research	
		Total Research	% of Total Research	Total Research	% of Total Research
1960	189	163	86	26	14
1965	521	409	79	112	21
1970	698	488	70	210	30
1975	1,465	859	59	606	41
1980	2,543	1,659	65	884	35
1981	2,662	1,838	69	825	31
1982	2,711	1,906	70	805	30
1983	3,007	2,182	73	825	27
1984	3,411	2,488	73	924	27
1985	3,930	2,900	74	1,030	26
1986	4,043	3,042	75	1,001	25
1987	4,816	3,589	75	1,227	25
1988	5,167	3,804	75	1,303	25

Source: *AAMC Data Book* (1990), Table I2.

SUMMARY AND CONCLUSIONS

The major support for medical research in the United States is the NIH. Now more than 100 years old, this federally financed institution is the largest biomedical research center in the world and by far the largest provider of financial support to biomedical researchers throughout the United States. As one of several components of the DHHS, the NIH enjoyed a budget appropriation of $8.3 billion in 1991, 88–90% disbursed in the form of competitive grants to researchers in U.S. schools, hospitals, and research institutes throughout the 50 states and the remainder devoted to biomedical research on the NIH campus.

Congressional appropriations to the NIH have increased (in constant dollars) almost every year since 1940. The allocation of these funds extramurally has varied greatly among traditional research projects, centers, contracts, and training agents. At last count, the funding of investigator-initiated research projects had risen to 66% of extramural award monies, and training grants had fallen to 5%.

The 13 Institutes of the NIH vary widely in their disease-oriented missions and staff sizes, in their individual appropriateness from Congress, and in their priorities for extramural awards. The Warren Magnuson Clinical Center, with its nearly 500 beds and extensive outpatient facilities, is dedicated to bedside research that cannot be undertaken effectively at other research sites. The staff members of the 13 Institutes who utilize these facilities have no teaching responsibilities and offer no medical services to the general public. Only patients who fit the research objectives of these physician-scientists are invited to share the facilities of the Clinical Center and are admitted free of all charges.

7

NIH Support of Biomedical Research

The modern era of the NIH began at the end of World War II, when Dr. C.J. Van Slyke, head of the Office of Research Grants of NIH, was charged with two responsibilities: (1) disposing of the war-time research contracts between the country's biomedical scientists and the OSRD and (2) establishing a new and expanded program of extramural research grants and fellowships. This infant program, which awarded $850,000 in 1946, has grown into an NIH giant (the Division of Research Grants, DRG), the first step in a two-step reviewing process that in 1988 disbursed nearly $5 billion to biomedical scientists throughout the United States.

The NIH takes understandable pride in having devised an effective process for reaching decisions on research applications. To ensure fair play and to minimize federal bureaucratic controls, Van Slyke set up a system of initial review groups (IRGs) that are staffed exclusively by extramural experts. As congressional appropriations for biomedical research swelled in size, so did the number of applications for these funds and the number of IRGs reviewing them: In 1989 more than 140 IRGs were responsible for reviewing more than 25,000 competitive applications. More than 2,000 extramural experts are engaged each year in this peer review process: during their 4-year terms of appointment, they travel to Bethesda for 3 days three times a year to review the applications assigned to them—an assignment that costs each of them at least 6 weeks of preparation time each year. That expenditure of time and effort is repaid by the educational experience gained in that pro bono service, and by the collegiality of working intensively and cooperatively with one's peers.

FEDERAL SUPPORT FOR RESEARCH AND ITS CONSEQUENCES

The consequences of accepting public funds were not analyzed by recipients as long as those funds were abundant. Indeed, from the end of World War II to the early 1960s, the federal purse seemed to have no bottom: not only did the number of medical schools and teaching hospitals increase, but research laboratories grew even more strikingly in number, size, and sophistication. The pursuit of medical science was so widespread that those not engaged in it found themselves swimming outside the mainstream: research (and the federal money supporting it) became the engine driving the schools and dominating their cultures.

It may seem incredible that anyone would have questioned the worthwhile-ness of accepting these lavishly proffered funds, but in 1951 Herbert Gasser, MD, Nobel Laureate and director of the Rockefeller Institute for Medical Research (now Rockefeller University), noted in his annual report to the members of the Institute's corporation that the

> shortcomings of the grant system are easy to see. They follow directly from the two conditions: projects and limited terms. In order to receive aid an individual must outline a project. At the outset he is in effect asked to make a prediction. Faced with this impossibility he may out of caution set his sights too low. *Projects, by definition, are not consonant with free inquiry* [emphasis mine]. At best they become obstructions for a good man to circumvent, as he makes his way. At worst, in the scramble for support, they may be devised with one eye upon the objectives of the donor, and without regard to whether the problem is at present ready for solution—an extraordinarily futile procedure when beset with a time limit. A tendency arises for the direction of research to be guided by the sources of funds, rather than by the uninfluenced initiative of the investigator. Through the limited terms of the grants, continuity is based entirely upon hope for renewal. Thus, there is a lurking inducement to engage in short-range enterprises so as to have something to show "when the term is ended."

These prescient words were delivered at a time when the Rockefeller Institute lived entirely on its endowment: outside grant money was never sought until Detlev Bronk succeeded Gasser as president of the Rockefeller Institute in 1953. In driving the transition of Rockefeller from a research institute to a post-graduate university, Bronk encouraged his rapidly growing faculty to apply for these newly available federal research funds. (Currently, about 50% of its operating budget is derived from federal sources.) Gasser also said that

> admittedly the grant system is highly effective in the promotion of research, and there is no gain-saying that accomplishments of the highest type can come out of it in spite of its shortcomings. . . . It is possible to see the aspects of scientific production which will flourish well. Development of all new leads that appear will be expected. Planned research, director-centered and organized with duties for a large number of workers, will be given the chance to show what it can accomplish. Mass explorations with known methods will yield useful additions to information. And problems requiring the gathering of statistical data will progress.

However, after the mid-1960s, the Golden Goose no longer laid enough eggs to satisfy the demand: seemingly unlimited access to research funding became a fond memory. The honeymoon years of biomedical science gave way to other realities when the vast social changes of the 1960s (and the federal funds demanded by these social needs) were recognized and heeded.

When in 1979 Wyngaarden tolled the bell for biomedical scientists in an

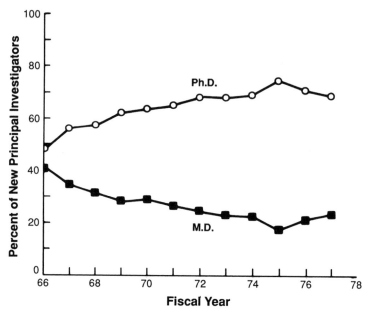

Fig. 7–1 New PIs on NIH research projects by type of earned degree. (Wyngaarden, 1979, Fig. 6)

article with the catchy title "The Clinical Investigator as an Endangered Species," his physician-scientist audience knew exactly what he meant, and they were easily persuaded that "the enemy is us": the proportion of NIH grants awarded to MDs had been falling over the previous 10 years, while those to PhDs had risen, and the proportion of new PIs who were MDs and MD-PhDs had fallen from 40 to 25% (Fig. 7–1). Wyngaarden's message: MDs are losing the race for grant funds to PhDs because "of a failure of the MD investigator pool to grow at the same rate as that of the PhD pool."

The validity of the conclusions drawn from such numbers and the implications of these trends will be examined in detail later. Suffice it to say here that the morale of aspiring young investigators declined noticeably during the 1980s and sank to a new low in late 1989, when the word got out that, at the last round of awards for grant applications, the success rate had dropped to 10–15% [a news story by Joseph Palca in *Science* (Nov. 24, 1989) was titled "Hard Times at NIH."]] To get to the root of the problem, we must look at the process by which a research application travels on its way from high hopes to money in the bank.

By focusing attention on the NIH process, I do not overlook the importance of private sources of research funding (foundations and individual donations), for such sources have been and will always be critically useful. But the magnitude of private, non-federal, non-profit funding, though it reached nearly $750 million in 1988, is overshadowed by the immensity of NIH funding for research, which outweighs it nearly 10 to 1. Nor can we overlook the contributions of industry, which grew from 29% of the national support for health R&D in 1979 to 45% in 1989. Although industry contributes important research funds to investigators in academic settings, there is no official tally of this contribution; and it is the common perception that most industry research money is spent within its own walls, and much more on D than on R.

THE NIH AWARDS SYSTEM

The NIH encourages the submission to it of proposals of many sorts—from small-business innovations to construction grants—but the most important research grants (for biomedical research in general, but especially for the salvation of any endangered species) is the traditional research project, coded as RO1 in the *DRG Activity Codebook.* RO1 grant awards made up 54% of the dollars awarded for all sorts of extramural applications in FY1988, whereas PO1 grants (program projects involving multiple disciplines and many investigators in addition to the PI) drew down 13%, and research centers (offering expensive resources to be shared by many departments and investigators) 12%.

It is the RO1 application that we will now track, but the general principles guiding the review of all NIH awards are the same. All are competitive, peer reviewed (but in various ways), and funded through one (rarely more than one) Institute, with annual budgets and time limits clearly spelled out in the award statement. No matter how many extramural scientists and other personnel are paid on any one NIH grant, there is only one PI per grant; and all transfers of funds are made not to PIs personally, but to the institutions in which they are employed. All NIH awards consist of direct cost allowances for salaries, permanent equipment, supplies, travel, and publications costs, but also of indirect cost allowances for administration, energy, security, library, and custodial services. Thus, direct costs support the research intentions of the PI, while indirect costs are paid to meet the overhead costs of the institution in which the PI works.

Allowances for indirect costs are set by local "cognizant federal auditing agencies" that adjudicate the claims of each institution at least every 3 years. Indirect costs are computed either as percentages of all direct costs or as percentages of wages and salaries; these percentages vary widely among the several types of extramural awards made by the NIH, from low rates for training grants (8%) and for off-campus research (33.5%) to 65% or more for RO1 grants. In FY1989 the total expenditure by NIH for indirect costs amounted to 46% of direct costs; indeed, over the last 10 years, the rate of increase for indirect costs has exceeded that for direct costs because of growing numbers of federal regulatory requirements for safety, affirmative action, drug-free workplaces, and so on, as well as rising costs for energy needs, waste disposal, security, library needs, custodial services, and administrative costs.

Writing the RO1 Application

The applicant (MD, MD-PhD, PhD, or any other post-graduate degree holder) selects a scientific question that he considers important and soluble with the tools and skills at his disposal. The design of the experiment is thrashed out with his mentor (if he has one), and the writing begins.

There is a standard format for the RO1 application: The face page of Section 1 provides a wide variety of identifying data about the project, the applicant, the nature of the institution in which the project will be pursued, whether the appropriate approvals have been obtained from local institutional review boards for involvement of human subjects or vertebrate animals in the research plan, total costs (both direct and indirect), and signatures of officers of the institution certifying their agreement to comply with all relevant federal regulations.

On the second page, the applicant presents a brief synopsis of the long-term objectives and specific aims of the project, as well as the experimental design and methods for achieving these goals. On this same page, the applicant must also list all key personnel engaged on the project.

Pages 3, 4, and 5 itemize in detail the proposed budget for the first year, and for all subsequent years up to a maximum of 5. Justifications of the budgetary requests for all personnel costs, costs of unusual items, and reasons for budget increases after the first year are requested.

The rest of Section 1 is devoted to biographical sketches of all key personnel, limited to two pages each; a complete itemization of all other sources of budgetary support for all key personnel (no page limit); and a description of the physical resources available to the applicant (no page limit).

Section 2 begins with the Research Plan (limited to 20 pages): the specific aims (usually one page or less), background of the study and its significance (2 or 3 pages), studies performed by the applicant before filing this application (6–8 pages), and a detailed description of the experimental design and methods to be used.

Following the 20-page Research Plan, a number of pages (unlimited) are devoted to descriptions of all plans for involving human subjects and/or vertebrate animals, and evidence of compliance with all federal regulations dealing with human or animal rights or both. Biographical sketches of all consultants (2 pages each) and their letters of agreement to participate in the project come next, followed by a 4-page limit for all current and relevant bibliographic references cited in the Research Plan.

A final Checklist certifies compliance with eight federal regulations dealing with employment rights, misconduct procedures, freedom from federal debt, absence of debarment or suspension by any federal agency, presence of a drug-free workplace, and absence of all lobbying activities on behalf of the applicant or the application. The Checklist closes with a detailed rendering of indirect costs and how they were calculated.

Applicants, if they wish, can also submit an appendix (unlimited number of pages), "photographs, oversized documents or materials that do not photograph well," pertinent to the project but supplementary to the essentials contained in the 20-page limit of the Research Plan.

The instructions for completing this RO1 application are 23 pages in length; they conclude with the following statement: "the Public Health Service [PHS] estimates that it will take from 10–15 hours to complete this application—which includes time for reviewing the instructions, gathering needed information, and completing and reviewing the form." This astonishingly low time estimate by the PHS is certainly not shared by investigators throughout the country, but I know of no hard data to support the anecdotal evidence (and my personal experience) that writing an acceptable RO1 application requires at least 50–100 hours. At least 30 pages are required for an RO1 application (25 for the text alone); most applications exceed 50 pages if they are filed by an applicant working with two or three key personnel.

Wise applicants ask for their colleagues' reactions to the proposal before mailing the complete package (original and six copies) to DRG. There are three deadlines each year for receipt of RO1s (and other types of applications), at which point a given application begins its way through the review system: The minimum time from receipt by the DRG to the earliest payment date by one of the Institutes is 10 months.

Referral of Research Applications to Reviewing Bodies

Research applications of all types are received by the DRG and logged in by its Referral Office, from which they are distributed in many directions by a seasoned staff of readers. Applications are of three types: new, continuation, and supplemental. Continuation applications are of two sorts: those that are annual reports submitted during the ongoing term of an award (these are not competitive and hence are forwarded only to the funding Institute), and those that are submitted at the end of a term award as applications for continued funding. Since the latter group of continuation applications compete with all new applications, they must be sent to one of the IRGs. Finally, supplements to existing awards can be requested: they are also competitive and must be reviewed by one of the IRGs for scientific merit. Table 7–1 shows the numbers of these three types of awards in FY1988; competing awards made up 34% of all research grants awarded, and 70% of the money went to grants approved in previous years.

At each of the three deadline dates for receipt of applications in the DRG offices, rooms are piled high with applications to be sorted according to the nature of the research proposed. The Referral Office staff reads each application and designates it for two sequential levels of review: first, to the most appropriate IRG and, second, to the particular awarding component (Institutes, Centers or Divisions, or ICDs) whose mission is most relevant to the objectives of the application. When questions arise regarding the optimal routing pathways, advice is sought from the executive secretaries of the DRG's Study Sections or of the ICD's Review Groups to ensure the most knowledgeable hearing for each appli-

Table 7–1 NIH Research Grants by Type in FY1988

	Number of Grants in FY1988 and Annual Growth Rate (1979–88)[a]		Amount in FY1988[b] and Annual Growth Rate (1979–88)[a]	
	No.	Growth Rate	No.	Growth Rate
Total	26,023	3.3%	$4,727,320	10.3%
Type of Grant				
New[c]	4,974	1.6	655,239	8.0
Continuation				
Competing[c]	2,977	2.9	709,729	9.5
Non-competing	17,158	4.2	3,285,386	11.2
Supplemental[c]	914	−1.7	76,965	6.4

[a]Calculated from Table 26, *NIH Data Book* (1989).
[b]Dollars in thousands, from Table 26, *NIH Data Book* (1989).
[c]Competing applications.

cation. Thus, the Referral Office of the DRG is a triage site that is swamped three times a year with applications that must be logged in, their receipt acknowledged, and their initial assignment made either to the ICD's Review Groups (about 20% of all competitive applications) or to the DRG's Study Sections. (The DRG reviewing process and the relationships between the DRG and the various Institutes of NIH are described in detail in a 200-page reference and training manual: *DRG Handbook for Executive Secretaries*, August 1990. The specific areas of interest within each of the DRG and ICD review groups are detailed in the *DRG Referral Guidelines for Initial Review Groups of NIH*, 1989.)

It is important to understand the basis for this important routing decision. The ICD's Review Groups handle all multicenter and multidisciplinary applications, program project applications, center and core grant proposals—in short, the large-dollar applications. From time to time the ICDs will issue Requests for Applications (RFAs) to deal with topics that they consider ripe for consideration by extramural applicants; the responses to these RFAs are automatically routed for review to ad hoc review groups of the requesting Institute. Applications for large clinical trials also are sent to the most appropriate ICD for review; nevertheless, these and the RFAs are coded as RO1 applications. In contrast, applications reviewed by DRG study sections are, in general, couched in the language of a particular scientific discipline and are smaller in their dollar requests than the applications routed to the ICD review groups.

In 1989 the 50 ICD review groups reviewed 5,010 competitive applications, of which 1,109 were subsequently coded as RO1s. That same year, the 72 chartered study sections of DRG, plus some 21 temporary, non-chartered study sections, reviewed 24,111 competitive applications, of which 16,665 were RO1s. Table 7–2 shows a comparison of the several types of research grants that passed through these two pathways of review and their numbers in FY1988.

Not shown in Table 7–2 are the following: 90% of all RO1 applications, and 90% of all RO1 award dollars, were initially reviewed by DRG study sections.

Table 7-2 Competing NIH Research Applications in FY1988, by Review Process (IRGs) and by Kind*

Routed Through the DRG Review Process	Number of Applications
A. R&D grants	
1. Traditional projects (RO1)	15,131
2. Recognition awards[a]	88
3. Post-doctoral career enhancement awards[b]	2,194
B. Research fellowships (F series—individual awards—mainly F32)	2,607
C. All other research[c]	3,069
	23,089
Routed Through the ICD Review Process	
A. R&D grants	
1. Traditional projects (RO1)[d]	1,593
2. Program projects (PO1)	473
3. Research centers[e]	411
4. Recognition awards[f]	556
B. Research training (T series—institutional awards—mainly T32)	624
C. Research fellowships (mainly F31 and F32)	400
D. All other research[g]	1,742
	5,799

*Kinds of activities. See *DRG Activity Codebook* for letter and numerical designations of these awards.

[a]Includes R37 MERIT awards and K01 Research Scientist Development awards.

[b]Includes R23 New Investigator awards (terminated in 1990 in favor of R29 FIRST awards) and K04 Research Career Development awards.

[c]Includes P41 Biotechnology Resource grants, R15 AREA awards, R22 U.S.-Japan Cooperative Medical Science programs, R43/44 Small Business awards, S10 Shared Instrumentation grants, and other R&S awards.

[d]Includes responses to RFAs.

[e]Includes G12 Minority Research Centers, M01 General Clinical Research Centers, P50 Specialized Centers, P51 Primate Research Centers, and other P awards (P20, P40, P42, P60).

[f]Includes all types of K awards, but mainly K04 Research Career Development awards, K07 Academic/Teacher awards, K08 Clinical Investigator awards, K11/12 Physician Scientist awards, and R35 Outstanding Investigator awards.

[g]Includes C06 Construction, G07/08 Library Improvement awards, G20 Repair grants, R03 Small Grants, R13 Conferences, R18 Demonstration Projects, R24 Resource-Related Research Projects, R25 Education Projects, S06 Minority Biomedical Research Support, U01 Research Cooperative Agreements, U10 Cooperative Clinical Research agreements.

Source: *DRG Peer Review Trends, Member Characteristics, 1977–86*, updated by personal communications with Lucille Nierzwicki, Suzanne Fisher, and Jo Ann Wingard (all of DRG).

The award rates (number of applications actually funded) were 28% for the RO1s reviewed by the DRG process and 23% for those passing through the ICD process; on the other hand, the average award dollars were $152,000 for the former group of awards and $190,000 for the latter. Thus, a lower proportion of RO1s was awarded through the ICD process, but at a 25% higher funding rate.

Study sections of the DRG are made up of some 15 to 20 non-federal scientists serving 4-year terms (one of whom is appointed chairman by the DRG) and an executive secretary who is a full-time health science administrator in the DRG, almost always a PhD by training. Applications referred to one of the 100 or more study sections of the DRG are mailed out to all members of that section by its executive secretary, who (sometimes in consultation with the chairman) designates two of the members as primary and secondary reviewers of each application and two more as "discussants." The wisdom and experience of the executive secretary are critical in making judicious assignments and expediting the handling of the workload at each meeting to ensure each application a fair hearing.

The primary and secondary reviewers bring to the meeting their written appraisals of the application and read them to the group. While all members of study sections are expected to read all the applications to be considered at a given meeting (at least a 2-week job before each meeting), the primary and secondary reviewers' written opinions weigh heavily in determining the fate of each application, although in open debate the reactions of the two discussants and other members can at times modify or even overrule those written opinions. The pressure to complete the evaluation of as many as 60–80 applications at a given meeting can be intense, and the chairman must intervene to guide the process to completion without short-changing any of the reviews. With only 60 applications to process in 2½ days, each application gets an average of 20 minutes' consideration if the section works for 8 hours per day.

After each "case" is heard, the Section members record their confidential ratings, with 100 as perfect and 500 as poorest. (Outright disapprovals are few—less than 5% in 1988; they are not given a numerical rating.) After the meeting has been concluded, the executive secretary tallies the votes, and for each application a mean priority score between 100 and 500 is computed. Then all scores are re-computed on a percentile basis to indicate where each stands in comparison to the other grants reviewed at that session. This way, each grant gets two ratings: a priority score and a percentile rating.

The percentile rating allows comparison of one study section's ratings with another's. For instance, Study Section A may judge that its applications are so worthy that their priority scores all fall between 100 and 200, while Study Section B, reading their applications with a more sanguine eye, awards scores between 100 and 400. The percentile rating system rank-orders the scores of the two study sections in such a way that their ratings in relation to each other are comparable.

After all scores have been computed, the executive secretary frames a report to each applicant summarizing the views and conclusions of his section members, citing the strengths and weaknesses of the proposal, as well as the two scores. These summary statements (called "pink sheets") are mailed to the applicants as soon as they have been completed, even before all applications from the 100 or so study sections are re-sorted for forwarding to the Advisory Councils of the 13 Institutes for the second level of review and final decisions on funding.

Three times each year, the Advisory Council of each Institute receives as many as 500 competitive applications, together with the summary statements resulting from the first-level review. It is the responsibility of each Council to consider whether a given application fits the scientific mission of that Institute: it looks hardest at the large-dollar applications and attempts to minimize any duplication of awards; it also pays special attention to the minority and geographical distributions of its awards. In most cases, the IRG recommendations prevail. Finally, each Council determines what the payline (cutoff point) will be for that round of applications, based on the funds available in that Institute for extramural awards. Then all award statements are sent to the extramural institutions responsible for the conduct of that research, with a copy to each applicant stating whether the application has been funded or not, and at what dollar level.

The available funds at a given Institute may permit them to pay only those applications that rank, for instance, in the most favored 15% (specifically, with percentile ratings of 15% or lower). In that hypothetical case, all applications with percentile ratings of 16% or higher will be marked "approved but not funded." Since the funds available in the various Institutes vary greatly in any given year, their separate paylines will vary; thus, applications with a percentile rating of 25% or less may be funded by one Institute, while another Institute may be able to fund only those applications with percentile ratings below 15%.

Applications "awarded but not funded" can be re-submitted for consideration at the next round of IRG meetings if changes aimed at the criticisms noted in the pink sheets are made quickly (a process called "amendments"). Alternatively, they can be rewritten and submitted later as revised grant applications. An analysis of the "eventual success of first-time applicants" over the years 1976–88 (Robert Moore, DRG, November 1989) showed that 31% of MD and PhD applications were successful on their initial review; after first and second reviews, the success rates were 38% for MD's and 39% for PhDs; and after 5 successive yearly reviews, the rates were 46% for MDs and 47% for PhDs. (During those 12 years there were no significant time trends in these eventual success rates of MDs and PhDs.) While these data are not as discouraging as many young applicants seem to believe, it cannot be overlooked that some 55% of first-time applicants fail to win awards for a given research proposal, even after trying for 5 successive years.

Approval, Award, and Success Rates

At this point, it would be wise to define terms that are commonly confused. We have already distinguished priority and percentile ratings; now we consider approval rates, award rates, and success rates, as the NIH uses these terms.

"Approval rates" are the proportions of all applications submitted that are approved by IRGs (whether DRG- or ICD-affiliated). In recent years, approval rates have regularly exceeded 90%, indicating that almost all applications are judged to be acceptable in presentation and scientific merit.

"Award rates" are the proportions of all approved applications that are actually funded. In 1989 the overall award rate for research projects by all NIH components (all ICDs) was 29.4%, and for 1990, 25.3%. (Award rates differ from one Institute to another because of differences in the amount of money available for extramural grants among the several Institutes.)

"Success rates" are the proportions of all applications submitted and reviewed that are actually funded. In 1989 the success rate was 27.5% (because the approval rate in 1989 was 93.5%, and 93.5% of 29.4% = 27.5%).

We will discuss the time trends in these various rates later.

Reasons for Poor Ratings in Priority Scores at the DRG Study Section Level

Even though more than 90% of all research applications submitted to NIH are judged to be meritorious from the point of view of the applicant's scientific objectives, skills, and facilities, the IRGs naturally find some applications to be more appealing than others. What weaknesses among the approved applications result in poor ratings?

Cuca (1983) analyzed this question with an in-house group of five DRG colleagues by reading the pink sheets (summary statements) of disapproved applications and others most poorly rated. Her list of defects is usefully compared to the review criteria on which DRG Study Sections are advised to score the scientific merit of each application:

DRG Review Criteria	Cuca's Defects (in Order of Prevalence of Defects)
1. Significance and originality of the proposed research	1. Technical methodology (66%)
2. Appropriateness and adequacy of the experimental approach (methodology)	2. Weakness of research hypothesis (47%)
3. Qualifications and experience of the applicant and staff	3. Weakness of data collection procedures (41%)
4. Availability of needed resources	4. Inadequate study population and controls (40%)
5. Apropriateness of budget and duration of support	5. Inadequate data management and analysis (31%)
6. Animal and human rights protection	6. Lack of significance of the research problem (30%)
	7. Inadequacies of the applicant (17%)
	8. Inadequacies of the needed resources (4%)

Cuca reviewed some 2,000 applications that had recently passed through 13 DRG study sections and selected 256 of those with poor priority ratings for analysis with the help of five colleagues (three executive secretaries and two members of the Research Analysis and Evaluation Branch of DRG). The selection process was limited to applications involving patients or volunteers, excluding those dealing with in vitro studies of materials of human origin and those involving sociologic surveys. Thus, the Cuca study confined itself to clinical research Categories 1 and 2, excluded Categories 3 through 7 and all non-clinical applications, and paid no attention to comments on the budgets or on the human/animal rights aspects of the applications. By far the largest number of defects were tallied against the criterion called "technical methodology" (Cuca's criterion 1). (Cuca's criteria 1, 3, 4, and 5 are actually subdivisions of the second DRG review criterion.)

Cuca intentionally excluded all non-clinical applications (she called them "basic research applications") but compared her 1983 findings on clinical applications to three previously performed analyses that examined applications of all kinds. No significant differences were noted in the frequencies of the defects detected in earlier studies and those described above, so that "the reasons for disapproval and poor priority scores of clinical research applications [as defined by Cuca] seem to be essentially the same as those for basic research applications" [as defined by Cuca]. Cuca also analyzed her sample in terms of the highest post-graduate degree of the applicants (i.e., MD, MD-PhD, or PhD) and found "no significant relationship between the frequencies of types of shortcomings and the training/degree of the investigator."

In summary, then, methodologic weaknesses were the most common defects cited by DRG study section reviewers in the applications most poorly rated. In regard to defects, however, no real differences between applications submitted by MD and PhD applicants were noted, or between clinical and non-clinical applications.

Training Grants and Fellowships

Training grants and fellowships are applied for and reviewed in different ways. Institutional grants for training young MDs in various subspecialties (called "T32 grants" in the *DRG Activity Codebook*) are large-dollar awards that are rated by the review groups of the ICDs, rather than by DRG study sections. In contrast, "F32 fellowships" are applied for by individuals and are reviewed through the DRG study section process. T32 grants are awarded on a competitive basis to medical schools and teaching hospitals, which in turn choose for support those individuals who seem most promising in the eyes of their department chairmen. The records show that most awardees have spent a year or less on this form of support, during which they have learned various specialized aspects of patient care in a given subspecialty; the vast majority of these trainees has gone into practice and not into research. Nevertheless, this has been an important breeding ground from which to select the small number who choose to pursue academic careers and who achieve the degree of recognition that suggests to their seniors that they deserve to be supported henceforth as fellows (rather than trainees).

The most promising young MDs are encouraged to submit F32 fellowship applications in their own names (not as institutional designees). These applications are initially routed by the DRG Referral Office for competitive review by a study section set up specifically for review of fellowship applications in one of six broad disciplinary areas of biomedical research, and secondarily to the most appropriate awarding Institute. Other prestigious awards to young investigators also pass through the DRG study section review process, such as FIRST awards (R29). It is very clear that the DRG study sections play a crucial role in deciding who will be trained for clinical research and, subsequently, who will be funded. In due course we will examine the characteristics of these gate-keepers and how they have changed over time.

The Key Role Played by the DRG

In summary, then, the grants system of NIH is a complex mixture of applicants, procedures, and responders serving the many objectives of the biomedical research community. Because NIH awards come out of tax dollars, the grants system operates under certain constraints not borne by private, nonprofit agencies, but in size and number, NIH extramural funds are 10 times more abundant than those available from private sources. The importance to young investigators of winning RO1 support cannot be overestimated because of the importance assigned at every U.S. medical school to the NIH peer review process. Indeed, the RO1 grant to individual applicants is the backbone of the NIH awards system, consuming 54% of all NIH extramural award money in FY1988. We will see now how these awards have grown over time, to whom they have been made, and for what purposes.

TIME TRENDS IN THE AWARDS OF THE NIH GRANTS SYSTEM

Total NIH Obligations and Their Distribution

In FY1988 Congress appropriated some $6.6 billion to NIH for distribution to its four functional elements: Institutes and Research Divisions, the National Library of Medicine, the Office of the Director, and Buildings and Facilities. Table 7–3 shows this distribution, with 83% of the funds devoted to extramural awards and 11% to intramural research in the (then) 12 Institutes. Of the $5.5 billion awarded extramurally, 85% went to research grants, 9% to R&D contracts, and 4% to research training. The annual growth rate in total federal obligations over the period 1979–88 was 8.5%, well above the rate of inflation (6.8%). The growth rate for contracts fell well below that of inflation, as did that for research training. The distribution to the Office of the Director over this 9-year period varied greatly (from $20 million in 1979 to $115 million in 1986 and down to $62 million in 1988), so that its annual growth rate shown in Table 7–3 is meaningless.

Table 7–3 NIH Obligations by Function/Mechanism in FY1988

		Amounts		
		$ in Thousands	% of Total	Annual Growth Rate (1979–88)
Total		6,610,430	100%	8.5%
Function/Mechanism				
1. *Institutes and Research Divisions*		6,461,985	97.8%	8.5%
R&D grants	4,669,870		70.6	10.3
R&D contracts	496,993		7.5	1.6
Research training	238,954		3.6	5.8
Cancer control	69,682		1.1	−0.01
(Subtotal)		5,475,499	82.8%	
Intramural research	715,039		10.8	8.4
Res. mgt. and supp.[a]	271,447		4.1	6.4
2. *National Library of Medicine*	67,700		1.0	5.9
3. *Office of the NIH Director*	61,716		0.9	13.5
4. *Buildings and Facilities*	19,029		0.3	−5.3

[a]Research management and support = management of extramural programs and Institute directors' offices.
Source: Table 8, *NIH Data Book* (1989).

Allocations of NIH Extramural Awards to Four Major Activities

The distribution of extramural awards in FY1988 is shown in Table 7–4, along with the growth rates over the period 1979–88 in amounts and numbers of awards. Among the amounts distributed through the four funding mechanisms—grants, contracts, and training (two types)—none kept pace with inflation except for R&D grants. For all four mechanisms, the annual growth rate in number of awards fell well below the growth rate for dollars awarded, indicative of increasing costs per award over this period (for more detail on this, see below). Thus, while the growth in dollars for research grants may seem encouraging to some extramuralists, the absolute decline in individual training awards should be a source of concern for the long-term prospects of biomedical research. The annual trends in dollar awards from 1979 to 1988 for the four major activities is shown in Fig. 7–2.

These changes reflect the decision by the several Institutes of NIH to encourage awards to investigator-initiated research projects and to cut back on contracts, resource centers, and special grants. The decline in "targeted research," as this latter type is called, and the increase in investigator-initiated research—the former generated by intramural forces and the latter by extramural initiatives—are presented in Table 7–5. The peak of one and the nadir of the other

Table 7–4 NIH Extramural Awards by Funding Mechanism in FY1988

	Amount in 1988[a] and Annual Growth Rate[b] (1979–88)		Number of Awards in 1988 and Annual Growth Rate[b] (1979–88)	
	Amount	%	Number	%
Total	$5,538,075	8.8	—	—
Funding Mechanism				
R&D grants	4,727,320	10.3	25,754	3.3
R&D contracts	565,094	1.9	1,252	−4.7
Research training				
Individual awards (F series)	45,033	3.9	1,944	−1.4
Institutional awards (T series)	200,628	6.1	1,404	1.2

[a]Dollars in thousands and number of awards from Table 21, 1989 *NIH Data Book*; these dollar amounts do not correspond precisely to those in Table 8, 1989 *NIH Data Book*, for reasons not explained.

[b]Calculated from Table 16, *NIH Data Book* (1989).

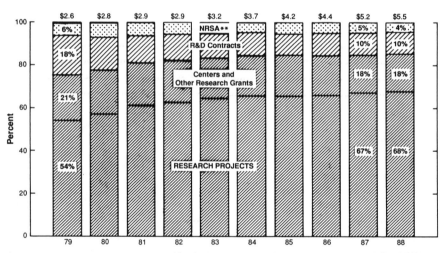

Fig. 7–2 Allocation of NIH extramural awards by activity, FY1979–88 (in percentages of total amounts awarded, current dollars in billions). (*DRG Extramural Trends, FY1979–88*, p. 6)

occurred in 1975, with reversals in directions thereafter. For the 3-year period 1986–89, the proportion for investigator-initiated research awards stabilized at 75% of total research dollars.

It should not be overlooked that in 1960—in the midst of the golden era of NIH funding—targeted research awards made up only 14% of total extramural award dollars. Then, over the next 15 years, perhaps due to pressures on Congress and the NIH for research of direct health benefit to the public, the propor-

Table 7–5 NIH Support of Investigator-Initiated vs. Targeted Research[a] (in Millions of Current Dollars)

FY	Total Research Dollars	Investigator-Initiated		Targeted	
		Total	% of Total	Total	% of Total
1960	189	163	86%	26	14%
1965	521	409	79	112	21
1970	698	488	70	210	30
1975	1,465	859	59	606	41
1980	2,543	1,659	65	884	35
1981	2,662	1,838	69	825	31
1982	2,711	1,906	70	805	30
1983	3,007	2,182	73	825	27
1984	3,411	2,488	73	924	27
1985	3,930	2,900	74	1,030	26
1986	4,043	3,042	75	1,001	25
1987	4,816	3,589	75	1,227	25
1988	5,167	3,804	75	1,303	25

[a]Targeted research = contracts, resource centers, and special grants.
Source: Modified from Table 12, *AAMC Data Book* (1990).

tion of targeted extramural research awards nearly tripled, reaching 41% of total awards in 1975. These changes produced a general hue and cry on behalf of so-called basic research, with a resultant decline in targeted (applied) research awards. Clearly, there can be no magical "best balance" between targeted and non-targeted research: As times change, research directions, opportunities, and challenges inevitably change. A best balance in any given year is better left to free-market forces of scientific inquiry than to centralized decision making (caveat emptor!).

NIH Awards to U.S. Medical Schools

It may come as a surprise to biomedical academics that in FY1988 only 52% of total NIH extramural award dollars were distributed to U.S. medical schools (including major teaching hospitals and basic health-science departments administered by these schools). The other 48% was divided among four other groups of performers. A mix of non-federal research institutes, non-profit hospitals, state and local hospitals, and for-profit research institutes received 25%; schools of arts and sciences 12%; public health and dental schools 7%; and other higher educational institutes 4% (*DRG Extramural Trends*, FY1979–88, pp. 78–79). These proportions have remained quite constant; from FY1979 to FY1988, the distribution to U.S. medical schools has varied between 51.2 and 52.3%.

However, among the 124 U.S. medical schools ranked in terms of the total federal research dollars they received, the top 40 won substantially higher approval rates for all competing research project applications over those years (1979–88) than did the schools ranked 41–80, and these in turn received higher approval rates than the final third, ranked 81–124. The same disparities were also noted in success rates (number awarded as a percentage of applications received). From FY1980 on, the success rates for the top 40 medical schools averaged about 40%, for the next 40 about 30%, and for the bottom 44 about 20%. Not only did the research-intensive schools file more applications than the others, but apparently their applications were judged to be of higher quality by the peer review systems (*DRG Extramural Trends,* FY1979–88, pp. 82–85). Potential applicants may not be aware that this rank ordering among U.S. medical schools depicts qualitative as well as quantitative differences in their schools' research activities.

Number of Applications and Awards

There has been a steady increase in the number of competitive applications for research projects since 1977 but a far less striking increase in the number of applications awarded. Figure 7–3 shows these changes up to 1987. In FY1988 the number of such applications reviewed was 19,205, with 6,212 awarded, down from 6,446 in FY1987 (*NIH Data Book,* 1989, Table 34). The annual growth rates tell a less alarming story: from 1980 to 1988, the annual growth rate in applications reviewed was 3.9%, and for those awarded, 3.3%. It would thus appear that, since 1980, the balance between supply and demand for research project funding reached a kind of steady state, but unhappily at only about 30%.

But these averaged data conceal the important fact that competing and non-competing applications vie unequally for dollars awarded. To demonstrate this point, Table 7–6 shows important differences in total awards for all kinds compared to new awards of all kinds. Since 1977, the percentage of new awards has averaged about 19%, with no apparent time trends. Thus, only about 20% of awarded dollars go to new applications. It is noteworthy that in FY1988 only

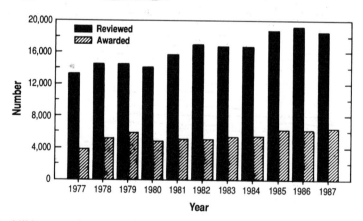

Fig. 7–3 NIH competing research project grants, FY1977–87. (*NIH Peer Review Committee Report,* 1988, Fig. 7)

Table 7–6 New NIH Grants in Competition for Funds with
Competing, Non-Competing, and Supplemental Applications
(1977–86)

FY	Total	New	% New
1977	15,564	2,602	16.7
1978	16,772	3,520	22.3
1979	19,204	4,307	22.4
1980	20,061	3,310	16.5
1981	20,418	3,168	15.5
1982	19,893	3,237	16.3
1983	20,819	3,842	18.5
1984	21,535	4,042	18.8
1985	22,958	4,703	20.5
1986	23,445	4,402	18.8
1987	25,026	5,153	20.6
1988	25,754	4,974	19.3
	Average % New (1977–88) = 18.9 ±2.31		
For 1988:			
Research projects (all)[a]	20,867	3,342	16.0
Traditional project research (R01)	16,871	2,230	13.2
Research centers[b]	621	51	8.2
Other research[c]	4,266	1,581	37.1
Totals	25,754	4,974	19.3

[a]Mainly R01, R43-44, R29 (FIRST), P01 (but also others) (see *DRG Activity Codebook*).
[b]Mainly P50, P30, P40 awards (but also others) (see *DRG Activity Codebook*).
[c]"Other research" includes Biomedical Research Support and Development awards, K awards, cooperative clinical awards, and minority biomedical support awards, plus a mix of some nine other kinds of awards making up 69% of new "Other research" awards in FY1988.
Sources: Tables 24 and 26, 1987 *NIH Data Book*, and Tables 26 and 28, 1989 *NIH Data Book*.

16% of all research projects were new and 13% were new RO1 awards, whereas in the case of "other research", much of which is Institute-generated, 37% of the awards were new.

Look now in greater detail at the award dollars for the three types of research projects: new, competing continuation, and non-competing continuation, and the changes in their proportions over the period 1978–88. As seen in Fig. 7–4, the largest proportion of award dollars supports non-competing continuation grants: In FY1988 the number of new awards of all kinds was 4,974, while the number of competing continuation awards was 2,977 (*NIH Data Book*, 1989, Table 26). These two categories of awards cost NIH some $655 million and $709 million, respectively, whereas the total dollar award for non-competing continuation awards was $3,285 million. This 2.4-fold difference is due to the large previous commitments for ongoing support of several years' duration to scientists whose applications had been funded prior to 1988.

It has long been evident that competing continuation applications (often

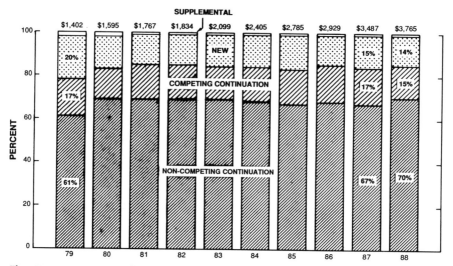

Fig. 7–4 NIH research projects by type, FY1979–88 (in percentages of total amounts awarded, current dollars in millions). (*DRG Extramural Trends, FY1977–88*, p. 22)

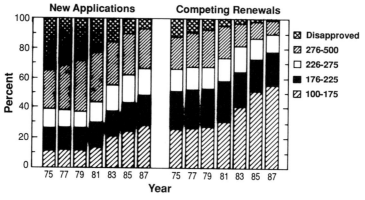

Fig. 7–5 DRG study section action on competing RO1 applications, FY1975–87. (*NIH Peer Review Committee Report*, 1988, Fig. 19)

called "competing renewals") enjoy higher priority ratings by the IRGs than new applications. This would be expected. Each of them has already been through the fire of peer review at least once, and thus, at renewal time, such applications achieve a better record of success than do new applications. This is graphically shown in Fig. 7–5 for the years 1975–87: While the disapproval rate for new RO1s fell from 35% in 1979 to 8% in 1987, it dropped from 12% to 1% for competing renewals. At the other extreme, the most favorable ratings (100–175) were bestowed only half as often on new applications as on competing renewals over this 12-year period. As a result, the award rate for new research project applications since 1982 (data not shown) has been a bit lower than 30%, but for competing renewals it has been more than 50%. To quote from *DRG Extramural Trends* (1979–88 p. 33), "Since competing continuations tend to receive better priority scores than new awards, and the payline(s) over the decade (have) dropped, more competing continuations are being funded in recent years, and the gap between the two has widened."

Award Rates of MD and PhD Applicants

The tables and figures presented so far in this chapter suggest that it can be a mistake to draw conclusions about the track records of MD and PhD applicants on the basis of the number of applications, because they represent a mixture of types of awards. First, it is misleading to lump all competing applications together, since the award rates for competing renewals are so much higher than those for new applications. It is even worse to lump together competing and non-competing grants: that practice aggregates three types of awards, all with different priority scores and NIH commitments.

Wyngaarden, sounding this alarm about "clinical investigators as endangered species" in 1979, described the declining number of MDs embarking on research training and subsequently qualifying as PIs on NIH research grants. He correctly pointed out that the declining percentages of NIH awards to MDs was due to the failure of the MD investigator pool to grow during the same years that the PhD investigator pool more than doubled. For example, he showed that over the previous 11 years the number of new MD PIs held relatively constant at about 300 per year, whereas after 1973 the number of new PhD PIs rose from about 500 to more than 750. In addition, he emphasized that the success rate of MD applicants was close to that of PhDs, indicating no disparity in the scientific value and editorial quality of the two kinds of applicants.

In 1988 Healy updated the numbers of NIH research grants awarded to MDs, MD-PhDs, and PhDs from 1970 to 1987 (Table 7–7) and proved again that the

Table 7–7 Numbers of All Types of NIH Research Grant Awards, Competing Plus Non-Competing (1970–87) (According to the Degree of the PI)

Year	Total No. of Grants	Number of Grants (% of Total)[a]		
		MDs	MD-PhDs	PhDs
1970	11,683	4,289 (36.7)	693 (5.9)	5,993 (51.3)
1975	13,899	4,485 (32.3)	797 (5.7)	8,017 (57.7)
1980	19,325	5,555 (28.7)	852 (4.4)	12,283 (63.6)
1985	22,271	5,807 (26.1)	808 (3.6)	13,725 (61.6)
1987	24,384	6,393 (26.2)	904 (3.7)	15,589 (63.9)

[a]The numbers shown do not add up to the totals (nor the percentages to 100), because a small number of other degree holders than those listed above also received grants.

Source: Reported by Healy (1988) and based on data supplied to her by the DRG, NIH, July 1988.

percentage of awards to MD applicants had fallen by nearly 30%, but she obscured the case by lumping together competing and non-competing grants of all types. To sharpen the comparison between PhD investigators and MDs as NIH grant winners, let us focus once again on that major NIH research grant, the RO1. Table 7–8 shows the number of new RO1 applications reviewed annually since 1970, the number of awards, and the success rates for MDs (including MD-PhDs) and PhDs. Note, first, that this table deals only with *new* RO1s. Thus, the total number of awards in any given year was far lower than the total shown in Table 7–7, due to omission here of non-competing and competing renewals. In the 1980s, the numbers of applications and awards to both groups of degree holders peaked in 1985, declining thereafter by 15–20% because of growing fiscal constraints. Since 1973 the number of MD applications has varied between 2,000 and 2,500 per year, while that of PhDs has risen from about 4,000 to more than 6,000 after 1977. Thus, the annual growth rates (1974–85) for PhD

Table 7–8   Number of New Traditional Project Grants (R01) Awarded (1970–88) (According to the Degree of the PI)

Year	Number of Applications MDs[a]	PhDs	Number of Awards MDs[a]	PhDs	Success Rates (%) MDs[a]	PhDs
1970	1,389	2,852	380	661	27.3%	23.1%
1971	1,480	2,806	458	737	30.6	25.8
1972	1,774	3,402	1,148	598	33.2	33.2
1973	2,057	4,012	460	770	22.2	19.1
1974	2,052	4,031	793	1,618	36.4	36.9
1975	1,982	4,377	695	1,765	34.8	39.3
1976	2,070	4,542	535	1,216	25.8	26.7
1977	2,246	5,836	517	1,284	22.9	21.8
1978	2,499	6,291	636	1,863	25.2	29.1
1979	2,505	6,924	796	2,422	31.3	34.2
1980	2,375	6,767	577	1,774	24.2	26.1
1981	2,481	6,639	579	1,595	23.2	23.9
1982	2,390	7,354	498	1,610	20.8	21.8
1983	2,308	7,150	553	1,800	23.9	25.1
1984	2,240	7,089	549	1,756	24.5	24.7
1985	2,489	8,011	588	1,992	23.6	24.7
1986	2,215	7,521	513	1,808	23.1	24.0
1987	2,036	6,378	516	1,679	25.3	26.2
1988	2,114	6,814	483	1,572	22.8	23.1
Averages (1970–88)					26.4%	26.8%
± S.D.					±4.60	±5.40

Annual Growth Rates

(1970–88)	2.4%	5.0%	1.3%	4.9%		
(1974–85)	1.8%	6.4%	−2.8%	1.9%		

[a]Includes MD-PhDs.

Source: Personal communication, Robert F. Moore, DRG, NIH (February 1989).

applications and awards were almost 4 times higher than those for MD applications.

However, as stressed in 1979 by Wyngaarden and in 1988 by Healy, the success rates of the two groups have been indistinguishable. The wide but coincident swings in these rates over time (note the large S.D.s) were most likely due to payline differences from one year to another. A final important lesson is to be drawn from these data: since success rates express the percentages of applications that are finally awarded, and since the success rates of MDs and PhDs were almost the same during the period 1970–88, the widely held perception that MDs wrote less sophisticated and less worthy applications than PhDs is simply wrong. The differences in the number of awards between these two groups have been due to differences in the number of applications filed, not to differences in their quality.

"Hard Times at NIH"

Even though the dollar appropriations to NIH by Congress have increased since 1979 at an annual rate of 8.5% (see Table 7–3), Joseph Palca, writing in *Science* (Nov. 24, 1989), said, "This has not been a good year to apply for a grant from the NIH. . . . In the fiscal year just ended, NIH funded only 29.3% of all approved projects competing for funds. That's an all-time low . . . and fiscal year 1990 will be worse."

While a number of reasons can be given for this situation, there is no doubt that underfunding has become a chronic condition, and one that must soon be addressed openly and seriously by the executive branch of the federal government, but also by a general population that will, in the long run, be under-served by its research community as health care problems persist and their costs continue to escalate. The concerns expressed by the biomedical community over this trend have become increasingly shrill. On that point, Kennedy (1990) includes an excellent piece of advice: "the scientific community should at all costs avoid any hint of endorsing the proposition that makes a research award look like an entitlement."

A major cause of the present NIH financial crisis is the fact that the indirect costs of research awards have risen even faster than the direct costs. Table 7–9 tells the story from 1970 to 1988: The average direct costs of research awards have increased almost fourfold in these 18 years (and faster than inflation), but indirect costs per award have risen more than sevenfold. Thus, in every way, it is costing more every year to support a PI's research. Salaries, wages, benefits, supplies and equipment, travel, and publication costs all have risen sharply as research technologies have increased in complexity, sophistication, and cost. But the overhead costs awarded to the institutions in which biomedical scientists carry out their research (heat, light, water, security, and administrative services), have risen even more sharply. In constant dollars, indirect costs have risen 114% from 1970 to 1988, while direct costs have increased only 15%.

Fixed costs ↑ sharply !

Table 7–9   Changes in Expenditures by NIH for New Traditional
Research Project Awards (R01)[a]

FY	No. of Grants Awarded	Average Cost per Award (in Current Dollars)		Average Indirect Cost Percentage[b]
		Direct	Indirect	
1970	1,101	26,724	6,195	23%
1971	1,774	29,360	7,490	
1972	1,872	32,074	8,718	
1973	1,206	36,409	10,136	
1974	2,537	40,434	12,382	31
1975	2,606	39,308	12,021	
1976	2,052	44,344	14,151	
1977	1,955	46,898	15,061	
1978	2,701	48,837	16,828	
1979	3,425	52,562	18,695	36
1980	2,512	58,551	20,852	
1981	2,399	64,325	24,112	
1982	2,261	68,714	26,762	
1983	2,574	69,320	27,779	41
1984	2,526	78,800	33,872	
1985	2,778	87,573	37,373	
1986	2,568	88,159	37,136	
1987	2,381	104,210	43,391	
1988	2,230	103,134	44,237	43
Annual Growth Rates (1970–88)	4.0%	7.8%	11.5%	

[a]Exclusive of expenditures by the Division of Research Resources and the National Library of Medicine.

[b]Indirect costs as a percentage of direct costs.

Source: Personal communication, Robert F. Moore, DRG, NIH (March 1988).

   Thus, the total costs per award in current dollars (direct plus indirect) have risen almost fivefold (data not shown), with an annual growth rate over those 18 years of 8.7%, which is well in excess of inflationary increases. The net effect of these disproportionate growth rates is that the various Institutes are unable to fund larger numbers of competitive grants each year, regardless of their scientific worth. As the direct and indirect costs per award increase faster than inflation, award rates must fall unless congressional appropriations rise to match the total costs per grant.

   A second major cause of the current funding crisis at NIH is due to a policy change among the Institutes in 1985 that was made in order to stabilize the scientific careers of their PIs: namely, to lengthen the duration of grant support wherever feasible and justifiable. Figure 7–6 shows that from 1977 to 1985, the mean duration of funding for competing RO1 awards hovered at around 3.25 years but then lengthened to nearly 4 years. (The wide ranges shown were due

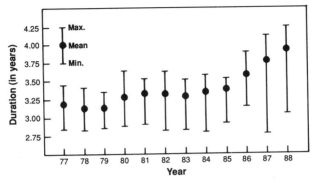

Fig. 7–6 Average duration of project periods for NIH competing RO1 Awards, FY1977–88 (with ranges of individual ICD averages). (*NIH Peer Review Committee Report,* 1988, Fig. 10)

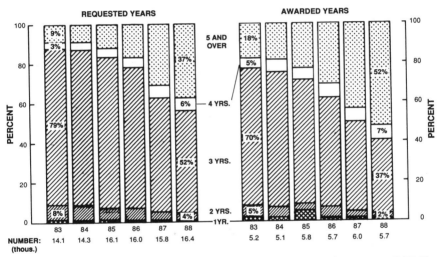

Fig. 7–7 Length of project periods for NIH competing research projects, FY1983–88. (*DRG Extramural Trends, FY1979–88,* p. 48)

to differences in priorities and paylines among the several Institutes.) Figure 7–7 looks at this phenomenon in another way: among the applications approved by the various IRGs, those recommended for approval for 5 years or more increased from 9% in 1983 to 37% in 1988. And of those finally awarded at the ICD level of review, the 5-or-more-year awards grew from 18% in 1983 to 52% in 1988. Three-year grants decreased to 37% of all awards. This has been welcome news for those PIs who formerly had to submit a competing renewal application only 2 years after receiving a first award.

Although this policy change has been applauded by the extramural scientific community, the consequence of this lengthened support period is that smaller amounts of the Institutes' funds are currently available for paying new awards.

This reason for the squeeze on funds will cease when the transition to longer award periods ends, but it is ironic that a change that has been welcomed by the award winners has obviously hurt those applicants whose ratings fall short of the various Institute paylines.

Action on newly targeted priorities such as research on AIDS and the human genome may have added to the current decrease in funds available for investigator-initiated research: $300 million for AIDS in 1990 and $58.5 million for the genome project. To what degree these costs are "new money" (that is, appropriated in addition to the already approved congressional budgets) is not clear. To the extent that these or any other new targeted research projects are drawn out of the total NIH appropriation (those cited come to only about 5% of the total NIH budget), there will be that much less money available for distribution to scientists engaged in research that does not enjoy such high priorities.

SUMMARY AND CONCLUSIONS

NIH awards for support of extramural biomedical research have grown from $850,000 in 1946 to over $5 billion in 1988, yet the demand for grant monies has exceeded the supply since the early 1960s, and seriously so in the last few years.

The process by which awards are made to extramural applicants is described in detail, using the traditional research project (coded RO1 by NIH) as an example: first, the nature of the application, and its processing through the NIH's Division of Research Grants to one of its 100 or more study sections for scientific review and evaluation of merit (the priority ratings); then the second review step by one of the Institute's Advisory Councils, and a decision for payment (or not) based on the funds available in that Institute at that time. At present, almost 95% of the RO1 applications are approved by the DRG study sections in terms of scientific merit, but less than 30% are actually funded due to insufficient funds at the Institute's levels.

More complex and costly research applications are forwarded to review groups within the Institutes for first-level review. Differences between the IRGs of the DRG and those of the 13 Institutes are spelled out in detail: both are made up of extramural experts, but the DRG groups serve 4-year terms, while those of the Institutes are often assembled for single ad hoc sessions. However, the latter groups are more senior and have more MD members who often serve repeatedly as reviewers. The workloads of the two review groups also differ, being five times heavier in the DRG study section process.

Training grants and fellowships cost the NIH about one-sixteenth the amount of money awarded for all other grants annually. These competitive applications also are reviewed for merit and fundability through the two-level process described for RO1 grants.

Time trends in these many different kinds of NIH awards are described in some detail, as well as two major reasons for the current shortage of funds despite increasing congressional appropriations to the NIH: (1) a 15% increase in the direct costs of each grant (in constant dollars) since 1960 but a 114% increase in overhead (indirect) costs, and (2) a significant lengthening of the duration (in years) of the individual grants to RO1 awardees since 1983. Both factors have seriously limited the funds currently available at each Institute for new awards of all types. At the same time, it is clearly evident that the success rates of MD and PhD applicants have been nearly identical for the last 20 years. Thus, differences in the number of RO1 grants to MDs and PhDs are due not to differences in the quality of the applications but to the number of applicants, PhDs outnumbering MDs by more than 3 to 1.

8

The Research Intentions of NIH Awardees

In Chapter 5 we described the size of the biomedical research establishment, with a major focus on the departments of medicine in U.S. medical schools and on the bedside research of physician-scientists at the NIH Clinical Center in Bethesda, Maryland. Consideration of the funding mechanisms for clinical research at these two very different work sites led us to a detailed description of the major funding source, the NIH, in Chapter 7, where we looked at the NIH system for awarding research grants, and at the trends over time in its record of research support for MDs and PhDs who have reached the status of independent investigators.

In this chapter, we shift attention from an analysis of the research *product* (the publications of researchers in Chapter 5) to the research *intentions* of young investigators and of older independent researchers who apply to the NIH system for research support.

Whatever the causes and wherever the solutions, extramural funding for biomedical research is sorely pinched. In this disheartening period of severe fiscal constraints, is it possible that certain types of research are doing better than others and that some types of clinical research are less endangered than others?

These questions could be answered if we had a more detailed understanding of the scientific objectives of young research-minded individuals who seek training in research methodologies and of others seeking early career support, and of still more experienced individuals who apply as independent investigators for RO1 grants. Throughout this search, we will persist in asking, "what kind of clinical research do these various groups intend to carry out?" This process will make it clear that of all the forms of clinical research, Basic POR is in the deepest difficulty.

RESEARCH INTENTIONS OF APPLICANTS FOR RESEARCH TRAINING AND EARLY CAREER SUPPORT

Physician scientist awards (K11) have been made since 1984 to newly trained clinicians nominated by their institutions on the basis of their interest in research careers and their perceived qualifications as promising investigators, but without prior research experience. These individual applications are competitively re-viewed by the review groups of the 11 Institutes and are awarded by the respec-tive Institute Councils. From 1984 to 1988, some 303 awards were made, and the 243 available abstracts of these awards were analyzed for their research intentions in the same manner as that described in Chapter 5 for research publi-cations. It was found that 30% of those 243 awards could be characterized as intentions to pursue some sort of clinical research, but only 7.4% of the total could be categorized as intentions to work on Basic POR (Category 1).

FIRST awards (First Independent Research Support and Transition awards) (R29) provide a sufficient initial period of research support for newly indepen-dent biomedical investigators to develop their research capabilities and demon-strate the merit of their research ideas. This award program began in 1986, and in FY1987, 588 of these awards were made via the DRG study section review process. A random sample of 199 of those awards was analyzed. Clinical re-search objectives were described in 41% of them, with 6% of the total sample categorized as Basic POR.

MERIT awards (R37), in contrast, are selected by the extramural staffs of 11 of the Institutes (the National Institute of Communicative Diseases and Stroke has a comparably prestigious award named the "Javits Award," which is simi-larly selected). These highly regarded awards are made to established investi-gators with extremely favorable priority ratings on their most recent competitive research grant applications. Established in 1986, some 596 MERIT awards were made through FY1988. All competitive 1986 and 1987 awards, numbering 335, were categorized in terms of the types of research in which these awardees were already engaged: non-clinical, 53%; Basic POR, 7.5%; and Categories 3 and 4, 32.9%.

The Kinds of Research that RO1 Awards Make Possible

Since 1973, the RO1 application form has required a specific "yes" or "no" answer to the question of whether, in any part of the studies described in the application, the applicant intends to involve human subjects (or any products derived from human subjects). If the answer is "yes," evidence must be given that the local Institutional Review Board (IRB) has given its approval of the intended work after assuring itself that the project fulfills all the ethical and safety requirements spelled out in the Code of Federal Regulations 45 CFR 46, Protection of Human Subjects (*Federal Register,* March 8, 1983), to protect the rights of human subjects engaged in research studies. If such an application is in fact awarded, the NIH database (CRISP) codifies that document as "human sub-jects" research.

Now it might be concluded that all human subjects applications deal with some aspect of clinical research and that all clinical research applications are coded as human subjects research. This, however, is not true. As already shown, much clinical research that does not involve human subjects and does not require IRB approval—for instance, animal models of disease and development of new technologies. Because of these semantic uncertainties, it became necessary to perform a survey of the RO1 grant awards individually in order to learn what each awardee intended to study, to see which review groups recommended their approvals and which Institute Councils actually made the awards, and to what extent clinical research is the exclusive province of MDs (or MD-PhDs).

In Chapter 5, we demonstrated that 36% of the 164 authors in the randomized 3-D Survey who published research reports in 1987–88 wrote one or more articles on non-clinical research, 86% one or more reports on some form of clinical research, and 39% one or more reports on Basic POR. In contrast, the CC Survey showed that in a sample of 33 highly selected physician-scientists at the NIH, 55% reported one or more articles on non-clinical research in 1988, 94% one or more articles on clinical research, and 67% one or more articles on Basic POR. On examining the distributions of research intentions among the PIs of new RO1 awards, we were surprised to find a number of striking differences from the above figures.

RESEARCH INTENTIONS OF APPLICANTS FOR RO1 AWARDS

The categorization process pursued in this RO1 survey was almost identical to that of the surveys described in Chapter 5, once the required RO1 abstracts were available for analysis. Each abstract was assigned either to non-clinical or to clinical research, and, if to the latter, to one of six categories. (In early 1988, when this study was undertaken, Category 6 was defined as a combination of two sorts of activities, development of new technologies and assessment of health care practices. In 1989, when the 3-D and CC Surveys were carried out, these activities were separated into Categories 6 and 7.) An appendix to this chapter describes the details of sampling and its representativeness.

The Categorization of New RO1 Applications

The assignment problem in this study was somewhat simpler than that in the 3-D and CC Surveys because, in this case, there were no book chapters, reviews, or case reports to consider, only the authors' abstracts and only one abstract per author. Although the editorial quality of the 557 abstracts varied considerably, they presumably represented each applicant's best attempt to furnish all the information needed for an informed reading by the reviewers on whose opinions the fate of the application so delicately hung. These 557 abstracts were assigned to one of seven categories—one non-clinical and six clinical research categories. The results of these assignments are shown in Table 8–1. In each target year, the actual numbers of awards in each of the seven subdivisions are given, as well as their percentages in the total sample. It is seen that from 1977 to 1987, the percentage of non-clinical awards declined from 49 to 40%, balancing the increases in clinical research awards from 51 to 60%. There were no discernible

Table 8–1 R01 Survey: Categories of Research Intentions in Random Samples of New R01 Grant Awards in Three Fiscal Years

	1977		1982		1987		All Years Combined	
	No.	%	No.	%	No.	%	No.	%
Classification of Awards^a								
Non-Clinical	94	49	90	45	68	40	252	45.3
Clinical	98	51	108	55	99	60	305	54.8
Cat. 1	15	8	16	8	10	6	41	7.4
Cat. 2	1	0.5	8	4	5	3	14	2.5
Cat. 3	22	11	18	9	18	11	58	10.4
Cat. 4	51	28	49	25	51	31	151	27.2
Cat. 5	3	1.5	8	4	11	7	22	4.0
Cat. 6^b	6	3	9	5	4	2	19	3.4
Total Clinical	192		198		167		557	

^aA total of 200 awards were randomly selected in each target year for analysis of their authors' abstracts; totals less than 200 are due to missing abstracts [The DRG database (IMPAC) included abstracts only after 1971.]

^bIn this survey, Cat. 6 included development of new technologies and assessment of health care practices. Some months after this R01 Survey was completed, Cat. 6 was separated into two parts: Cat. 6 (new technologies) and Cat. 7 (health care practices).

time trends among the six categories of clinical research over the 10-year span, except perhaps a small but consistent increase in Category 5 (field surveys).

The outstanding finding of this survey was the small size of the award rates for Basic POR (Category 1), averaging 7.4%. In contrast, the largest percentage of awards was made for research on animal models of human disease (Category 4), averaging 27.2%. Some experts have argued that research on animal models ought not to be considered to be clinical research at all, since that type of research does not deal directly with human subjects and is not so coded in IMPAC. However, in all 151 cases, the applicant named a specific clinical problem into which he was seeking new insights through research on an animal model; accordingly, I classified these abstracts as clinical research.

If the combined data for Categories 1 and 2, which deal with different types of studies in whole humans, are compared to the combined data for Categories 3 and 4, which are strictly laboratory studies, we see for the three target years the numerical dominance of laboratory-based research projects over those pursued through meticulous studies in human subjects.

	1977	1982	1987
Cats. 1 and 2	8.5%	12%	9%
Cats. 3 and 4	39%	34%	42%

Categories of Research in Relation to Postgraduate Degrees

The preferences for certain kinds of research by MDs, MD-PhDs, and PhDs were found in this survey to differ markedly from expectations, the most striking of which is the large number of PhDs engaged as PIs in clinical research. Table 8–2 shows an intriguing distribution of PhD to MD ratios among the several categories of research. While the largest number of PhDs are seen to have been PIs on non-clinical research projects, 45% of them (188) were PIs on clinical research projects. Even more surprising, the number of MDs and PhDs as PIs on Basic POR projects was almost equal (21 vs. 20).

This unexpected finding deserves further inspection and explanation. In terms of the distribution of Basic POR awards among the various Institutes, 18 of the 21 PhD awards were made as follows: by Child Health and Human Development (8), Eye (5), Heart and Lung (3) and Aging (2). In contrast, 17 of the 20 MD-PIs on category one research were awarded by Arthritis (9), Heart and Lung (5), and Eye (3). More revealing is a tally of the DRG study sections recommending their approvals. Basic POR awards to PhDs were almost all re-

Table 8–2 R01 Survey: The Relationships between Post-Graduate Training and the Pursuit of Various Research Objectives (Three Target Years Combined)

	Total Awards	PhDs	MDs[a]	% of Total Awards		
				PhDs	MDs[a]	Ratio
Total sample	557	418	139 (16)	75.0	25.0%	3.0
Non-clinical research	252	230	22 (3)	41.3	3.9%	10.6
Clinical research (all six categories)	305	188	117 (13)	33.8	21.0%	1.61
Basic POR (Category 1)	41	21	20 (1)	3.8	3.6%	1.06
Animal models (Category 4)	152	96	55 (8)	17.2	9.9%	1.74
The Universe[b]						
Total applications	27,272	19,568	7,704 (1,032)	71.8	28.2%	2.55
Total awards	6,341	4,573	1,768 (237)	72.1	27.9%	2.58
Success rates (%)	23.3	23.4	22.9			

[a]Includes MD-PhDs, with numbers of MD-PhDs shown in parentheses.
[b]The total number of applications and awards made by NIH in 1977 + 1982 + 1987.

viewed by study sections focused on social, behavioral, and developmental studies, sleep studies, vision, and communication research, whereas those to MDs were mostly reviewed by study sections of general medicine, metabolism, pathology, biochemistry, endocrinology and reproduction, pharmacology, and toxicology. Thus, MDs who were awarded RO1s for Basic POR totaled only 3.6% of the entire sample of 557 awardees, and for all 6 categories of clinical research only 21%!

The success rates for PhDs and MDs (Table 8–2 bottom) were nearly identical, one more indication of the similarity in science-worthiness of the applications of these two groups, as judged by IRG reviewers.

Comparisons Between the Output and the Aspirations of Physician-Scientists

The 3-D and RO1 surveys make possible an interesting comparison between what physician-scientists finally publish and what they intend to study if awarded grant support. Both surveys were carefully randomized, and they covered the same three time periods between 1977 and 1987. The following tabulation presents this comparison, in which the awards to PhDs in the RO1 survey have been deleted so as to focus on the RO1 awards to MDs and MD-PhDs only:

Research Applicants and Research Authors Compared (MDs and MD-PhDs only: Three Target Years Combined) (see Tables 8–2 and 5–8)

| | Applicants | | Authors | |
| | RO1 Survey | | 3-D Survey (Three Depts. Combined) | |
	No.	%	No.	%
Total number	139		164	
Non-Clinical Research	22	16	60	37
Clinical Research	117	84	141	86
Basic POR (Category 1)	20	14	55	34
Animal models (Category 4)	55	40	25	15

Note that the same high percentages of MD applicants and authors (84 and 86%) focused their research on clinical research topics. What is strikingly different, however, is the much lower percentage of MDs applying for research support for Basic POR (14%) than actually publishing it (38%) and the higher percentage aiming to concentrate on animal models of human disease (40%) than actually reporting on such research (14%).

Looking to the future, I find it ominous that less than 8% of the most prestigious early career awards made by the NIH and of new RO1 grants are aimed at Basic POR. In the 1950s and 1960s, this research activity dominated the pages of clinical research publications and the annual meetings of clinical investigators, but clearly, the pendulum has swung decidedly toward bench research (Categories 3 and 4) and away from Basic to Applied POR—i.e., from studies on the mechanisms of disease to studies on disease management.

The questions we must now address are these: Why is Basic POR waning in popularity and prosperity in the world of clinical research, and should anything be done about it? What part of this decline is due to today's fascination with exciting new reductionistic methods, especially in molecular biology? What part is due a diminishing number of Category 1 applications being submitted, and what part to perceptions of their lack of scientific merit by the IRGs of NIH?

Perceptions of differences in the quality of research applications clearly do exist, and in the next chapter we examine the role of peer review in the measurement of quality.

SUMMARY AND CONCLUSIONS

The research intentions of NIH awardees (for training and early career support and for new RO1 grants) have been analyzed by reading the authors' abstracts of their applications. Of the physician-scientist awardees (K11), 30% intended to pursue some type of clinical research, but only 7.4% described programs in Basic POR. Comparable percentages for FIRST awardees (R29) were 41% and 6%, and for MERIT awardees (R37) 47% and 7.5%. These three sets of analyses covered the years 1984–88.

The research intentions of new RO1 awardees were analyzed by selecting a random sample of 200 award statements in the target years 1977, 1982, and 1987. The representativeness of this sample was tested by four criteria and found to be acceptable. Although there was a small increase in the number of clinical research awards over time from 51 to 60%, the percentage of awards in Basic POR varied between 6 and 8%. The largest numbers of clinical research awards fell into Category 4 (animal models of human disease) at 27%, and 10% of the awards were made for in vitro studies of human materials (Category 3). PhDs captured 75% of all new RO1s, strictly in proportion to the number of their applications; that is, the success rates of MD and PhD applicants were almost identical. Of possibly prophetic importance is the fact that 45% of the awards to PhDs described projects in clinical research, and half of the Basic POR awards went to PhDs.

Comparing the research publications to the research applications of MDs (i.e., comparing the 3-D Survey to the RO1 Survey), 10 times as many MD authors published Basic POR articles as were awarded RO1 grants for Basic POR. This represents an important change in attitudes toward clinical research by MDs over time, with a shift in emphasis from Basic POR to animal models of human disease.

APPENDIX: RANDOM SAMPLING OF RO1 AWARDS

As in the 3-D Survey, three time periods were selected for analysis: 1977, 1982, and 1987. In each of these years, a random sample of *new* RO1 award statements (stratified by Institute), 200 in each year, was selected by Robert F. Moore, DRG, NIH. Using this sample of selected project numbers, a printout from the IMPAC database was then made that included the title of the application, the name, address and degrees of its PI, and the PI's complete abstract. Also identified were the awarding Institute, the IRG that had approved the application, the first-year dollar award, and the notation "Human Related" (or not, as the case might be). Each abstract was followed by a list of "descriptors" (chosen by trained readers in the DRG referral office) that catalogued many of the characteristics of the proposal; these descriptor lists often proved helpful in quickly surveying the content of the abstracts.

The Universe, the Sample, and Its Representativeness

The total numbers of new RO1 applications awarded by NIH in the three target years (the three "universes") were 1,954, 2,255, and 2,368. Thus, the sample sizes of 200 represented 9.8, 8.8, and 7.0%, respectively, of each universe, and since these percentages were so similar, it was not considered necessary to adjust the sample size to the three universe sizes.

The representativeness of these samples was tested in several ways:

1. *By awarding Institute:* Knowing the total number of new RO1s awarded by each Institute in each target year and the number of awards assigned to each Institute in each sample of 200, a statistical test (Wilcoxon rank-order test) was applied to these pairs of numbers for each target-year. The fit was perfect at each time period, indicating that none of the Institutes had been slighted in the sampling process.
2. *By percentage of human subjects awards:* In all target years combined, the percentage of human subjects awards was 31.1% of the combined universes and 29.7% in the combined samples.
3. *By percentage of MDs, MD-PhDs, and PhDs:* For the three universes combined, the percentage of MDs was 24.0% and that of MD-PhDs 3.7%; for the combined samples, the percentages were: MDs, 22.0%, and MD-PhDs, 2.9%.
4. *By total costs per award:* In each target year, the first-year award costs per grant (in current dollars) in the three universes and three samples matched within 3%.

These tests of representativeness are shown in more detail in Table 8–3. It will be noted that the sample sizes did not all come up to the 200 originally

Table 8–3 Representativeness of the R01 Survey: The Universes of New R01 Awards in 1977, 1982, and 1987 Compared to the Random Samples Drawn from Those Universes

	1977		1982		1987		All Years Combined	
	Universe	Sample	Universe	Sample	Universe	Sample	Universe	Sample
New R01 awards	1,954	192	2,255	198	2,368	167	6,577	557
Percent of human subjects awards[a]	29.1	24.9	29.9	32.0	34.0	32.5	31.1	29.7
Cost per award (current dollars)	61,766	60,255	95,454	96,975	146,010	141,705		
PIs								
% MDs	27.2	28.6	23.1	19.2	22.2	18.0	24.0	22.0
% MD-PhDs	4.4	3.6	1.9	0.5	4.8	4.8	3.7	2.9
% PhDs	68.4	67.7	75.0	80.3	73.0	77.2	72.3	75.0

[a]Human subjects research requires approval by local IRBs; such applications were not so coded into DRG databases until 1974.

intended. The reason for this is that in 1977, eight award statements lacked abstracts; in 1982, only 2 of 200 selections were missing; but in 1987, 33 abstracts were not yet on file. Accordingly, the percentages shown in Table 8–3 were computed on the actual, not the intended, sample sizes. The proportions of the various degree holders in the samples drawn were close but not perfect fits to those in the respective universes in the three time periods.

9

Peer Review and the Measurement of Quality in Biomedical Research

If quality could be measured with any degree of precision or reproducibility, choices would be easy—be they choices of medical school admissions, or residency selections, or awards for further training or for grant support, or selections of scientific articles for publication. Lacking that quantitative precision, we have come to rely on consensus seeking—reaching agreements by gathering the opinions of individuals with the greatest experience in a particular endeavor. What wins is what pleases the hearts and minds of most of the experts.

In biomedical science, consensus seeking is carried out in two intimately linked arenas: the publication of research results and the evaluation of grant applications and, in their first derivatives, faculty appointments, and selections of prize winners. These two peer review processes are carried out somewhat differently, but with the same subjective personal determinants.

The *publication of research results* calls on a formal but usually anonymous process of peer review—namely, an editor's gathering of the viewpoints of several researchers working in the same field, in which value judgments are presented by mail in writing. Reviewers are asked to comment on the importance of the work, its originality, the strength of the experimental evidence, the clarity and economy of the presentation, and its relevance to work already reported by others. If the editor finds a consensus among two or more reviewers on the acceptability of a submitted report, it will be published. And if the reviewers request revisions, the author has the option of making the changes or proving to the editor that they are not warranted. When all disagreements are reconciled, the report goes to the printer.

Such is the process in peer-reviewed journals—a process that can take a year or more for reports submitted to the most rigorous journals. A report that is published in a peer-reviewed journal is considered to have met certain criteria of quality and to have merited a stamp of approval that is important to the journal's readership.

As a measure of the quality of research articles, peer review can be said to be, at best, a highly subjective process, but one in which objectivity is the goal. Despite its inherently "soft" endpoints, this process is held in high regard because it is on publications that promotions, salaries, tenure, elections to prestigious societies, and prizes depend. Despite the many criticisms leveled at it, it is the best system so far devised, but as a process that plays so important a role in all scientists' careers, it deserves to be closely monitored, criticized, and revised.

"Bibliometrics" is a relatively new technology that attempts to evaluate the impact of the contributions of scientists to knowledge in a given area. Because scientists perceive differences in the prestige of one journal in relation to another, they tend to evaluate each other on the basis of their choice of publication outlets. Thus, bibliometrics starts by evaluating the merits of individual journals in which authors publish and the impact of a given journal on its scientific readership as measured by its page numbers per year, its frequency of publication, and the size of its subscription list. Then it calculates the impact of a given report on the work of other scientists by counting the number of times that report is cited in the publications of those other scientists. In these ways, the "soft" subjective process of peer review is given a "hard" ring of objectivity by setting up numerical indexes at several levels of peer review: the clarity and economy of an author's writing that makes it publishable, the choice of a journal in which an author publishes his results, the esteem in which that journal is held, and the number of times the work is quoted by other scientists in their own reports.

Bibliometrics is not intended to be an improvement on or a modification of editorial peer review. It is a complex enumeration of the various components of peer review, and its ring of precision has brought it considerable recognition as an important methodologic advance. Although bibliometrics gives a high gloss to the imprecisions of peer review, it is of questionable value in judging an *individual's* scientific merits. In the words of Francis Narin (1983), a chief practitioner of bibliometrics, "these techniques are eminently reasonable and powerful for the analysis of the *aggregate* scientometric properties of large laboratories and institutions, [but] they are at best of very limited utility when used in the analysis of the productivity of individual research scientists."

The evaluation of grant applications by peer review differs from editorial peer review in being a face-to-face committee process rather than an editor's collation of a small number of written viewpoints, but it too is a subjective process. One thing is certain: it is the keeper of the gates through which all RO1 applicants must pass. Let us look now at the nature of peer review at the NIH and the history of changes in it in recent years.

THE NIH PEER REVIEW PROCESS

When C.J. Van Slyke assumed responsibility for the World War II OSRD contracts in medical research in 1946, he dealt with a total of 66 contracts (later called "contract grants," then "grants") and a total budgetary obligation of $870,000. In 1947 his budget had grown to $4 million for extramural grant support, and in order to deal with its distribution, he enlisted the aid of 250 extramural scientists organized into 21 study sections. Today, as we have seen, the extramural grants obligation is over $5 billion, and there are more than 200 advisory boards, councils, and IRGs engaged in the evaluation of nearly 30,000 applications for research awards each year through the voluntary services of more than 2,000 extramural biomedical scientists.

To be invited, as I was in the mid-1950s, to join an NIH study section was a considerable honor—a sign of recognition that academic researchers covet. I joined with some 15 other so-called experts in metabolism and nutrition (as our section was called). Our meetings in Bethesda were intoxicatingly pleasant and instructive. Drawn from all areas of the country, we became firm friends and took pleasure in work that was considered a duty but also a privilege. We learned from each other in meetings that began early in the day and ended long after dinner with talk about this extraordinary new process for expediting research. Travel costs with a meager per diem allowance for food and lodging were paid by the NIH; we took for granted the need to live in double rooms at the least expensive rates, and sometimes we broke even financially. When the workload grew to exceed 120 applications per meeting, the section split into two, but the discussions of each application were usually constructive and rarely adversarial. The funds available to applicants seemed endless, and it was gratifying to be part of a rapidly growing national research enterprise. It was, nevertheless, a great deal of work to serve as a study section member—at least 6 weeks' work each year—but it was gladly volunteered.

A final nostalgic note: the generally accepted objective was to support promising scientists, on the premise that innovative people can be counted on to generate fresh new research ideas. What the scientist with a tested track record of research success proposed to do—the proposal, the general program of research, the "theme"—was read seriously and closely scrutinized; this was one way in which section members educated themselves and each other. And young investigators with no track record as yet were treated kindly; the originality of their proposals was the determining factor.

The squeeze on funds that began in the early 1960s has changed this situation completely. As the supply of funds had decreased, demand has increased, and the tenor of peer review, formerly low-keyed and constructive, has become more strident. The atmosphere of study section meetings is less generally educational because its members are so highly specialized. And the basis for decision-making has swung decidedly toward a hard-nosed assessment of the likelihood of successful performance of research protocols and away from a hopeful evaluation of the innovative capabilities of applicants. Sad to say, it has become more and more difficult to recruit experienced working scientists to serve on NIH reviewing committees.

Selection of Members of IRGs

The awarding of public money for biomedical research has always been an openly competitive affair, and from the start in 1947, the aim has been to ensure fairness and to avoid the dangers of powerful cliques and "old-boy" favoritism.

Geographical considerations play an important role in choosing members to serve on study sections. The selection process is also heavily influenced by affirmative action policies on minorities and gender. The process has become more democratic, but the scarcity of minority scientists has made it difficult to meet the explicit quotas of the DRG administration. After screening for conflicts of interest, the final choices of new members are ratified by the NIH director. This is ordinarily a pro forma matter, but in the selection of members of Institute Advisory Councils, which must by law include a set number of lay members, there have occasionally been political pressures to contend with.

The choice of individuals for service on the IRGs and Advisory Councils of the Institutes is made internally at the NIH by the extramural affairs staffs of the Institutes, while those chosen for service as DRG study section members are made by the executive secretaries of the DRG. Most NIH staff members are scientists with a record of some years of research outside the NIH in one of the many biomedical research fields; the fact that they have chosen to accept staff appointments at the NIH would indicate that they have chosen administrative paths in preference to the increasingly insecure futures inherent in extramural research careers. The 100 or more executive secretaries and the 8 or 10 referral officers of the DRG are almost exclusively PhDs (with a few MAs), as are the staff members in the Offices of Extramural Affairs in the various Institutes.

Who are these key choice makers, and what are their qualifications? I know of no published evaluation of the scientific backgrounds of these important gatekeepers, nor of their performance records as NIH staff members. In striking contrast, the characteristics of the members of the DRG's study sections are spelled out in exquisite detail each year, as well as the trends in their performance over the years. In addition, there are voluminous annual listings of the names, addresses, and scientific interests of all extramural consultants to NIH (see NIH Advisory Committees, 1989, and *DRG Competency Roster of NIH Initial Review Groups,* 1988).

Before discussing the strengths and weaknesses of today's peer review system at the NIH, let us look at the differences between the two kinds of IRG's: those that serve the DRG and others that serve the ICDs.

1. ICD reviewers are older and hold higher academic ranks, and the IRGs of the Institutes have a higher percentage of MDs than do those serving the DRG. MD membership in DRG groups fell from 46% in 1977 to 30% in 1987; for the ICD groups, MD membership over the same period decreased only slightly, from 59 to 53% (*DRG Peer Review Trends, Member Characteristics, 1977–86,* pp. 13 and 97; *DRG Extramural Trends FY1979–88,* pp. 13 and 97).

2. Fifty percent of ICD review group members serve more than once, compared to 10% of DRG members. The reason for the low re-enlistment to DRG study sections is the commonly held belief that being a section member handicaps that member's own applications. The DRG says that this is not the case; such applications are reviewed by a section other than that of the applicant member or by a special study section called for ad hoc review of that application. The section members rebut by stating that this practice produces a less sophis-

ticated assessment of their applications by review groups lacking continuity in the process of decision-making. (It was once the custom for a section member merely to absent himself from a meeting in which his own application was under discussion, but this is no longer done.)

On the other hand, since study section members are chosen on the basis of their competence and experience, it is no surprise that the applications of present and former section members earn more favorable priority ratings and higher award rates than those of other applicants (*DRG Peer Review Trends, Member Characteristics 1977–86*, pp. 64–65, 70–71).

3. In the ICD system, many review groups are convened on an ad hoc basis, with members meeting on a single occasion to evaluate the responses of extramural applicants to specific scientific proposals advertised by the Institutes these are called: "Requests for Applications (RFAs)" and "Requests for Proposals (RFPs)." In contrast, DRG reviewers meet three times a year for up to 4 years, thus establishing an important degree of continuity in decision-making. DRG groups can invite ad hoc consultants to attend a given session in order to fill a gap in the scientific expertise of that meeting, and occasionally special study sections are called up by DRG for ad hoc meetings on applications addressing topics outside the realm of the regular study sections.

4. The workloads of the two sets of IRGs are far from comparable in terms of the numbers and types of applications they review. The DRG groups work under greater pressure of larger total numbers of applications, whereas the ICD groups review a more varied mixture of applications with higher individual cost commitments (see Table 7–2).

5. The appraisals of applications among discussants at ICD groups are more leisurely and more general in scope, and more members participate in them. In a small recently reported study of IRG behaviors, Scheirer and Garringer (1990) found that DRG groups expended less discussion time per application: 85% of the applications were discussed for 7 minutes or less, compared to 7 minutes or more for 56% of the ICD applications. In the DRG groups, fewer than 25% of the members engaged in discussion of 60% of the applications, while in the ICD groups, more than 75% of the members discussed more than 90% of the applications.

Strengths and Weaknesses of the NIH Peer Review System

The NIH peer review system is seen as one of the jewels in the NIH crown. Its main virtue is fairness to applicants whose appeal for research support is judged, not by a dean or a committee of intramural colleagues or by self-perpetuating boards of trustees of small foundations and private corporations, but by constantly rotating groups of nationally recognized experts who are external to the source of the funds, the NIH itself. At its best, the process is constructive in its critiques and advice to applicants; it is reasonably expeditious in terms of reaction time; and the process can be fulfilling for its reviewers.

The most valuable and perceptive analyses of peer review are those of Ingelfinger (1974), Horrobin (1982), Lock (1985), Bailar and Patterson (1985), and Stossel (1985). Criticisms of peer review in the grants world are of three types: those directed at the process itself, at the qualities of the study section members, and at the performance of the executive secretaries. In regard to the process, the workloads are too large, time is too short, and the endurance of reviewers is often exceeded. Because the basis for reaching judgments on applications has shifted in recent years from the accomplishments of the applicants to the details of the proposed projects, there is less risk-taking by applicants in describing their plans and more emphasis on accepted methodologies. It has been complained that these changes represent increasing attention to the *procurement* of research results at the expense of *investments* in scientific productivity—the same complaint lodged by Gasser in 1951 and quoted at the beginning of Chapter 7. Others (Finch, 1961; Luft and Loew 1980) have remarked on the increasing rigidity of the peer review process and on an increasingly adversarial atmosphere that looks more at the weaknesses than at the strengths of applications—what Osmond (1983) bitingly called the "decapitation" process.

The membership of current study sections also comes in for criticism: members are too young, too inexperienced, too focused on methodologic details at the expense of broader objectives, too self-protective, too caught up by a concern over old-boy networks. The most serious complaint, in terms of the future welfare of clinical research, concerns the selection of the MDs chosen for service on study sections. Not only are they shrinking in number—from more than 50% to less than 30% of the total DRG study section roster—they are also younger, less highly ranked in their academic faculties, and more likely to be narrowly reductionistic in training and in their own research endeavors.

Third, the executive secretaries are criticized for writing overly long, less accurate, and less knowledgeable summary statements (pink sheets). This is a serious charge, which, if true, frustrates the applicants who feel that their intentions have been misunderstood. One cannot help but sympathize with these overworked DRG staff members. With personal experience in one field of biomedical research, they must, nevertheless, cope with a variety of disciplines among their section members and among the applications as well. And the workload keeps growing.

In closing this topic, it is worth repeating the plea of several commentators that all components of the peer review process be continually evaluated and critically analyzed by a group of extramural senior scientists who meet periodically with a rotating panel of members, and not for single ad hoc sessions.

Peer Review Reviewed

There have been two recent studies of the DRG peer review process, the first an intramural panel report and the second a follow-up study by an extramural panel. The NIH Peer Review Committee, made up of internal NIH staff members and chaired by Claude Lenfant (director, National Heart, Lung, and Blood Institute), was appointed in 1987 by the NIH director (James B. Wyngaarden) to review all aspects of peer review in order "to improve the quality of the peer review system, making it more responsive to the scientific and administrative communities." Its report was filed in December 1988. Then a DRG Ad Hoc Panel of extramural scientists was set up by the Lenfant committee; it was convened in February 1989 under the chairmanship of Alfred P. Fishman (University of Pennsylvania). It divided into three working groups to consider three specific issues, then met in plenary session in November 1989 and filed its report in December 1989. (The recommendations of the Fishman panel aroused an extremely defensive response by DRG executive secretaries and review section chiefs, reported in June 1990.) The deliberations of these two reviewing groups and their recommendations can be considered together, since they resulted from inquiries and consultations made over much the same time period.

Recent Innovations

1. Applicants are now encouraged to suggest the study sections they consider most appropriate for review of their applications.

2. Amended applications are encouraged for rapid re-review of applications "awarded but not funded," provided that the revisions are clearly identified so that reviewers can quickly compare the old and new versions.

3. Seminars have been introduced as part of some study section meetings to broaden the scientific horizons of the members, many of whom are narrowly specialized. (This need for "focusing seminars" seems an implicit criticism of the disadvantages of the increasing diversity of skills represented in the membership.)

4. In addition to the usual designation of primary and secondary reviewers, extra discussants have been chosen in order to provide at least four informed opinions on each application. Written opinions are not requested of these discussants. (The need for discussants seems an implicit criticism of the diminishing thoroughness with which the applications are read by the section as a whole.)

5. Recruitment of experienced reviewers for duty on study sections has become a pressing problem that has been ameliorated somewhat by greater use of consultants. As a stopgap measure to meet a growing problem of recruiting full-term reviewers, a "reviewers reserve" has been created from which to call up experienced reviewers on an ad hoc basis.

6. The ratings awarded to each application secretly by each member of a Study Section have been a constant concern over the years because of differences in behaviors and viewpoints among the many Study Sections whose recommendations are directed finally to the (now) 13 Institute Councils. Raw averages of ratings gave way to normalized ratings, then to a trial of deletion of outlier ratings (at extremes of high and low approval), and most recently to a percentile system that was adopted "across the board" in 1988. Percentile ratings have

proven to be a convenience for the Institute Councils, which can now make a more equitable evaluation of the scorings of more than 100 Study Sections that funnel recommendations on more than 8,000 applications to them three times each year.

Studies Completed or Underway

1. Surveys have been made in five DRG study sections of the perceived importance of four criteria used by reviewers in reaching their priority ratings: concept of the proposal, competence of the applicant, design of the proposal, and the resources and environment in which the research is to be carried out. It was found that the reviewers on these five IRGs gave most weight to the research concept and protocol design, considerably less to the competence and track record of the applicant, and least to the resources and environment. However, the wide differences in opinions of the many members thus surveyed were far more impressive than the cohesiveness of their opinions (Lenfant report, pp. 8–11).

2. A test of review by mail was proposed by the Lenfant committee, and has recently been completed and reported by Scheirer and Garringer (1990). The purpose of this test was to ascertain whether mail reviews (the procedure followed routinely by the NSF) offered advantages over the present committee process. It was concluded that mail review was no less costly and no more effective that the present process. A total of 142 applications rated this way, in comparison to their customary handling in three DRG and five ICD review groups, attained essentially equivalent ratings when the opinions were averaged. (However, there were so many discordant judgments that the acceptability of *either* form of review might have been questioned.)

Major Unresolved Issues in Peer Review

1. The growing number of applications poses the most crucial problem for DRG staff and for study section reviewers. Although the average number of applications reviewed per meeting was 65, the differences among the various sections were very large, and in 1988 some 20% of the sections reviewed more than 80 applications. All who participate in the peer review process are overworked, and unless the number of applications is considerably decreased (or the number of reviewers and staff is increased), some deterioration in the quality and effectiveness of review must follow.

2. The Lenfant committee recommended (p. 17) that "reviewers be encouraged explicitly to pay careful attention to the qualifications and track record of the PI and associates in their assessment of the experimental approaches proposed." (This criterion has always been held suspect by young reviewers concerned over old-boy favoritism).

3. Innovative research suffers as award rates decrease, because "the peer review system encourages projects in the current mainstream of research and is biased against innovative research" (Lenfant report, p. 13). There are mechanisms in the NIH system for support of "innovative" research (although that term has not been carefully defined) and for pilot studies of new, untried research ideas (SO7 Biomedical Research Support Grants and RO3 Small Grants). The Lenfant committee looked with favor on the practice in some ICDs of setting aside a certain percentage of competitive dollars to be earmarked for the support of innovative research (p. 16) and to encourage creativity. While the committee noted that this has proved to be a workable mechanism, some of the Institute Councils are apprehensive. For instance, the designation of set-asides by Congress for specific purposes has sometimes resulted from public lobbying; this, of course, defeats the purpose of peer review and decreases the funds available for awards to competing grants.

4. The application process can be speeded up through the use of modern communication tools (Lenfant report, p. 25) and made less burdensome on applicants by imposing stricter limitations on page lengths and numbers of cited publications.

5. The perception that study section members are disadvantaged in consideration of their own applications has been considered false by the DRG itself, since the priority scores of such applicants have been consistently higher than those of non-members since 1976 (Lenfant report, Fig. 14). The DRG argues that during their service on study sections, the award rates of members did not exceed those attained prior to such service. This is taken as evidence that section members do not show favoritism in their ratings of other members. However, this argument has not proved convincing to the many study section reviewers who increasingly refuse to serve second terms. The Lenfant and Fishman panels urged that more definitive data be collected on the reasons given by prospective members for declining to serve on DRG study sections.

6. The question of the optimal size and number of DRG study sections remains open, with many of the Fishman panelists favoring more sections— smaller and more focused. The majority view, however, has endorsed the present system of large sections with a diversity of talents among their members. Those who object state that diversity itself undermines the collegiality of the group and allows the ratings to be too heavily influenced by the small number of members who are most familiar with the subject matter of a given application.

7. Both panels recognized the need to make DRG study section membership more attractive to the experts so badly needed. Not only has it become increasingly difficult to persuade such experts to accept these appointments, but the dropout rate of MD members who resign during their 4-year terms has tripled since 1976, from 4 to 14%, compared to a *decrease* in the resignation rates of PhDs from 10 to 7% (Fishman report, p. 32). These MD-resignation rates should also be viewed in terms of the greatly reduced number of MDs who accept appointments in the first place, from 44% in 1976 to 28% in 1984 (Fishman report, p. 32.)

Issues Not Addressed

1. There has never been a controlled experiment on the reproducibility of DRG study section reviews. In fact, Cole et al. (1981) found convincing evidence of non-reproducibility in the decisions of NSF reviewers when they submitted 150 NSF grant proposals to two different sets of equally qualified reviewers. They concluded that concordance in ratings appeared to be due to chance and suggested that success in NSF funding is due more to the choice of reviewers than to the substance of the proposal. The DRG has never reported a study to evaluate one set with another set of equally expert reviewers, both working in the same general field.

2. The expertness of the executive secretaries in assigning applications to their reviews, in absorbing the substance of the discussions about them, and in translating the written and spoken views about the strengths and weaknesses of the application to the applicants and to the awarding Councils has not been openly evaluated. How are these staff members chosen, and from how large a pool of applicants? How are they evaluated prior to and during their duty on study sections? What feedback mechanisms help them to perform their important duties increasingly well?

The Fishman panel report explicitly stated the necessity of superior performance by the DRG executive secretaries. It urged that they receive stronger administrative support in the form of well-trained technical grants assistants, updated computer equipment, access to library materials, and attendance at conferences inside the NIH as well as extramurally. In addition, the report expressed deep concern over their increasing workload. The executive secretaries, reading between the lines, took considerable offense at the Fishman report's implied challenge to their authority, as indicated by their response in June 1990. The fact that the viewpoints of extramural critics and intramural players are in conflict makes it even more clear that all differences of opinion deserve to be aired openly and periodically evaluated.

BOTTLENECKS: MONEY (SHORT-TERM) AND PEOPLE (LONG-TERM)

When funds for biomedical research were in ample supply, more than 70% of the applications submitted by extramural scientists were awarded. Academic freedom to pursue research goals was in evidence everywhere (perhaps to the detriment of medical school teaching, which came in a poor second in the faculty members' allocation of time and effort). And innovativeness was given full rein.

These conditions no longer exist. Funds for biomedical research no longer equal the demand for them (NAS-IOM Forum on Supporting Biomedical Research, 1990). With everyone aware that less than 30% of all applications will be funded, it seems to be the common perception that if an investigator just keeps filing one request after another, sooner or later one may reach the payline. The DRG toils harder and harder to process more and more applications that are filed by applicants who are spending more and more of their time writing more and more grant requests. Since the approval rate for these applications now exceeds 95%, the problem is not lack of clarity in grant writing or lack of wisdom in reviewing those efforts. It is simply the fact that there is not enough money in the Institutes' coffers to pay the growing number of acceptable applications.

These shortages at the Council level have only now begun to cause the biomedical research population to shrink. In these circumstances, it may seem futile to persuade more MDs to take up research careers and to spend years in training, only to end up writing multiple grant proposals. It seems equally futile to aim to improve the quality of grant writing, or to improve the DRG review system, unless radical changes in the entire process are adopted.

The advice given by one academic leader after another to MDs who want to pursue research careers is to get better research training in order to catch up to the PhDs. I cannot agree: MDs will spend valuable years attempting to catch up to PhDs who have spent all their post-college years acquiring laboratory skills and experience. Given the current shortage of funds, little will be gained except a sharpening of the competition between MDs and PhDs for available funds. Is increased competition worthwhile when alternatives exist?

It is gratifying that MDs and PhDs have, to date, been cooperating more fully with each other than ever before. Already there are many PhDs who, with the laboratory experience that MDs lack, have chosen to work on problems that are clearly designated as clinical research. Robust partnerships should be encouraged with these skilled PhDs, who since their college years have focused their efforts on one or another biomedical science during the 7 or more years that MDs have spent in becoming equally knowledgeable in the field of clinical medicine. The ability to recognize important medical research opportunities and challenges is the skill that MDs bring to such partnerships. Each partner should feel obliged to learn the language of the other in order to communicate optimally and to appreciate the full value of the other's background and skills.

This partnership cannot be achieved until the leadership in our biomedical institutions recognizes the need for it and establishes the secure career tracks in clinical departments for PhDs that rarely exist today.

However attractive this collaboration between MDs and PhDs may be in the short term, scientifically and fiscally, today's fiscal crisis in the funding of biomedical research cannot be solved by money alone. In the long term, we face a population problem, truly a Malthusian dilemma. Biomedical scientists have been reproducing themselves at such a rapid rate that the country can no longer afford to support their needs. I myself have been responsible for the early training of at least 30 young investigators over the last 30 years, and this is certainly not a record high. If every senior scientist "produces" one clone of himself each year, and if the productive "half-life" of each scientist is as little as 15 years of scientific research, it is inevitable that the researcher population will become so large that its demand for nourishment must eventually exceed the capacity of the system to supply it. That seems already to have happened.

The dilemma voiced 200 years ago by Malthus dealt with the imbalance between population growth and its food supply, but that concern has been allayed temporarily by advances in agricultural science and by the development of new food-distribution techniques. Conceivably, the current fiscal crisis in biomedical science can be met by severe rationing of supplies, equipment, and even people, so as to reduce the ever-rising direct costs of research. More acceptable would be to curtail the overhead costs of research by separating the overhead costs of administration and services to patients in our swollen academic health centers from the true overhead costs of research and teaching. But simply to infuse more money into the system, from whatever sources, will not solve the fundamental problem. It would not be long before an even larger population of scientists would be clamoring for still more financial support.

The realization of the odds against gaining support for a research career as brief as 10 years (or roughly three successes in winning a new RO1 and two competitive renewals) has already driven young investigators out of research (Movsesian, 1990). Clearly, it is fruitless simply to sharpen the competition for grants; we have already been so successful in producing large numbers of capable scientists that we are pricing ourselves out of the market. Completely new strategies must be sought with which to meet this extraordinary challenge. I have seen no evidence that the bases of this dilemma are understood by those in the strongest leadership positions; in a very recent position paper, Lederman (1991) argued against taking any positive steps toward what he called "scientific birth control," but his position is not persuasively defended.

SUMMARY AND CONCLUSIONS

High standards in the publication of research results and in the review of grant applications are sought today by different processes of peer review. Editorial peer reviewing involves gathering a few expert opinions on the worthiness of a given manuscript, usually anonymously and via the mails. In contrast, grant applications are evaluated in committees through face-to-face debate. A new technology, bibliometrics, assesses the apparent impact of the published contributions of scientists on knowledge in a given area of science; it does not pretend to be an improvement on the editorial review process. It is best used in evaluating the scientific output of large laboratories or institutions and is not appropriate in forming judgments of individual scientists.

The NIH evaluates the relative merits of the thousands of grant applications sent to it each year by peer review committee that answer either to the DRG or directly to the several Institutes. The compositions of these two peer review processes differ, as do their workloads and the types of applications processed by each. The DRG study section process has been studied and evaluated repeatedly; the ICD peer review process has not. Two recent reviews of the DRG process, one intra- and the extramural, have outlined its strengths and weaknesses, and have emphasized the critical importance of the executive secretaries of the 100 or more DRG study sections to the effectiveness and fairness of the system, and the increasing difficulty each has in coping with a growing workload of applications. (Surprisingly, there has been no published evaluation of these secretaries in terms of their scientific and managerial qualifications and their year-to-year performance.) Both reviews noted the need to make far more attractive the position of a study section member, especially to MDs who are increasingly declining the invitation of the DRG to join a section for a 4-year term.

Even if the process of peer review of NIH grant applications were faultless, it is now clear that the number of applicants for research support exceeds the supply of funds available now and very likely in the future. By training young investigators, scientists have reproduced themselves at such a high rate that the problem now is not the amount of the money for research but the number of well-trained people seeking it. With the passage of every year, the demand for funds by scientists will outstrip the available funds, so that the odds of gaining a succession of grants, even to make secure a 10-year career in research, are so low that young investigators are turning away from this career. This desperate Malthusian situation requires a complete re-thinking of strategies and research missions.

10

Sites at Which Patient Oriented Research (POR) Is Performed

The nature of POR has evolved dramatically over the last 150 years. The modern era began with purely descriptive studies that clarified the nature of human diseases and codified them into well-defined syndromes and disease entities. It then evolved rapidly through advances made possible by a succession of new technologies (bacteriology, physiology, biochemistry, and, most recently, molecular biology) that have allowed its investigators to employ increasingly sophisticated methods in their studies of man.

Today's enthusiasm for modern technologies need not diminish our admiration for the ingenuity of the POR investigators who succeeded in bringing medicine out of the darkness of mysticism and untested theory and into the bright light of empiricism, as brilliantly demonstrated by Claude Bernard in the 1860s. Today, when we gaze in awe at the 500-bed research hospital in Bethesda, Maryland, we should not forget the modesty of the circumstances in which Sir Thomas Lewis made such great strides in clinical research 60 years ago. Nor should we forget that exceptional advances depend only in part on the introduction of new techniques; more important is the curiosity, insights, and reflections of the investigators applying those techniques. As Gasser emphasized in 1951 (and many others before and after him), an innovative spirit is what most deserves to be nurtured.

The Hospital of the Rockefeller Institute for Medical Research, which opened its doors to patients in 1910, is thought to have been the first such facility devoted exclusively to research on human disease. Once the germ theory had been fully accepted in the late nineteenth century, the ferment for advances in medicine grew, and the need to bring science into American medicine stimulated the formation of the Rockefeller Institute and its unique hospital, led by Rufus Cole (Corner, 1964). It was Cole's objective to train a new generation of scientifically minded doctors through a novel combination of bedside and bench research on some of the most pressing medical problems of the day—syphilis, lobar pneumonia, poliomyelitis, heart disease, and "intestinal infantilism" (diarrhea of the newborn). Training physicians in science while providing the opportunity to discover—that was Cole's aim. It is an interesting coincidence that the

Flexner Report condemning the sorry state of American medical education also appeared in 1910. In different ways, Cole and Flexner were expressing the unrest and dissatisfactions of that era and voicing their hopes for change.

Only 3 years later, Lusk and Dubois established their unique metabolic ward in New York City's Bellevue Hospital and carried out their pioneering studies on energy metabolism in humans. At Boston's City Hospital, the Thorndike Laboratory, which adjoined the rooms of patients under study, was opened in 1923 under the aegis of the Harvard Medical School; this was followed by the establishment of Edsall's famous Ward 4 at the Massachusetts General Hospital in 1925 and the clinical research facility (Osler 5) at Johns Hopkins in 1930. These are only a few of the early sites for POR in the United States—all adding luster and intellectual excitement in their medical school environments. A growing army of clinical researchers listened with keen interest to the results of investigations on humans that were presented annually in Atlantic City, New Jersey, after 1911 and until these clinical meetings moved to other sites in 1979.

It was due to the farsightedness of Thomas Parran, Surgeon General of the PHS, that a research hospital was included in the 1944 legislation that created the NIH, but not until 1953 did that Clinical Center admit its first patient. It is said that the philosophy of the Clinical Center was modeled on that of Cole's hospital at Rockefeller, but its structure was at least 10 times larger. At the two sites (New York City and Bethesda) the aim was the same: "the physical structure of the [Clinical Center was] designed to facilitate cooperation and interchange between bench and bedside medicine; and access to the wide range of clinical and basic scientists on campus facilitate[d] cross-disciplinary advice and collaboration" (IOM, 1988a, p. 26). What was unique to the two institutions was that neither was involved in medical school teaching or community health care. The MDs who staffed those two POR sites could devote their entire energy to research, free from the time constraints of teaching and service.

However, aside from size, there are fundamental differences between these two POR sites. To quote the IOM report again, "The major advantage [of NIH] derives from financing that does not depend on discrete, time-limited grants or contracts awarded on a competitive basis" (p. 24). Although the Rockefeller Institute (now called Rockefeller University) was and is privately endowed, over the last 30 years it has become dependent on federal monies for support of its 50 laboratories, as well as for its hospital. At present, some 50% of the Rockefeller operating budget comes from research grants, mainly from the NIH—a process of intense national competition unknown *within* the NIH. But, on the other hand, "As a government laboratory the NIH intramural program is obliged to respond to congressional requests and national priorities that affect its scientific agenda. In practice, although Congress allows the program managers great discretion in establishing research priorities, there is a continuing, but beneficial tension in the appropriate balancing of congressional and scientific imperatives" (IOM, 1988a, p. 24). The NIH answers to Congress, and Rockefeller answers to the NIH!

THE NIH CLINICAL CENTER

Although familiar with the operating philosophy, facilities, and staff at the Rockefeller site, I nevertheless found it necessary (and illuminating) to look carefully into the workings of the NIH Clinical Center in order to compare its operation with that of other POR sites. I am indebted to John L. Decker, director of the Clinical Center, and to his staff for helping me to gain a deeper understanding of how the Clinical Center works, and to the deputy director for intramural research, J. Edward Rall, for permission to carry out confidential interviews in 1989 with each of the clinical directors of the (then) 12 Institutes.

At the top of the NIH hierarchy is the NIH director, who is, in more than theory, responsible to Congress for the performance of the several Institutes, each of which is headed by a director who oversees both the intra- and extramural programs of that Institute. Under each Institute director is a scientific director who is responsible for the quality of intramural science and the allocation of intramural budgets. In turn, the clinical director of each Institute is in charge of the facilities allocated in the Clinical Center to that Institute's clinical activities, but he answers to the scientific director on matters of the quality and costs of that Institute's bedside research. Except for the National Institute of General Medical Sciences (NIGMS) (which has no intramural science program), each of the other Institutes is made up of divisions, laboratories, and branches (in that hierarchical order), but only a few of these are involved in clinical activities. Most of these subdivisions are focused exclusively on laboratory research that is keyed to the congressionally mandated mission of that disease-oriented (categorical) Institute (see *DRG Referral Guidelines for Funding Components of PHS*, 1990).

Thus, the Clinical Center in 1990 consisted essentially of 12 hospitals, each with a different mission, each separately manned and budgeted. All of them are serviced by a central core of departments under the Center's director: surgery, pathology, rehabilitation, social service, intensive care, pharmacy, radiology, nutrition, nursing, blood bank, medical records, nuclear medicine, and housekeeping.

THE GENERAL CLINICAL RESEARCH CENTERS SCATTERED THROUGHOUT THE UNITED STATES

In 1959 Congress, inspired by its establishment of the Clinical Center, passed enabling legislation that authorized a country-wide distribution of small copies of the Clinical Center; these are called "general clinical research centers (GCRCs)." In 1960 the first centers were set up at a few prominent medical schools: Johns Hopkins University (Baltimore), Washington University (St. Louis), the University of Washington (Seattle), Emory University (Atlanta), the

University of Pennsylvania (Philadelphia), the University of Michigan (Ann Arbor), and the University of Southern California (Los Angeles). Each of these GCRCs (and others that were rapidly organized at others sites) was constructed in a location separate from the general wards and general out-patient clinics, with an organization like that shown in Fig. 10–1. The PI is typically a top official of the institution (dean, chancellor, vice-president for research, etc.), who testifies to the school's commitment of support for the center and to its agreement to adhere to all the rules and regulations dealing with research on human subjects. The program director, by contrast, is charged with day-to-day management of the GCRC under the watchful eye of an advisory committee composed of senior faculty members from pre-clinical and clinical departments. Patients are studied in special in-patient and out-patient areas, and occasionally in beds scattered throughout the general hospital; the four special units shown at the right of Fig. 10–1 support those studies. Investigators from all departments in the medical school are encouraged to utilize these facilities and to carry out their research studies there with the assistance of fellows and medical students. Research patients are carefully selected to suit the study needs of the user teams; they are admitted free of charge.

These GCRCs grew rapidly in number in response to demands for them, as indicated in Table 10–1, with a peak number of 93 centers in 1969 and 1970, and with funded beds exceeding 1,000 between 1965 and 1969. New and renewal applications for these centers have always been competitive on a national basis. They are awarded on the basis of the recommendations of an advisory

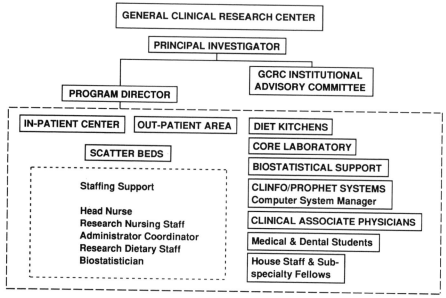

Fig. 10–1   Organization of a typical GCRC. (GCRC Program Evaluation, Phase I, 1989, Fig. 1; Dr. Judith Vaitukaitis, Director, GCRC Branch)

Table 10–1 Changes in the GCRC Program, 1960–89

Fiscal Year	No. of Centers	No. of Funded Beds
1960	8	133
1961	32	506
1962	56	760
1963	66	878
1964	77	994
1965	82	1,045
1966	88	1,097
1967	91	1,137
1968	91	1,070
1969	93	1,023
1970	93	904
1971	82	881
1972	84	907
1973	83	893
1974	87	877
1975	84	823
1976	84	784
1977	82	755
1978	79	633
1979	74	613
1980	75	602
1981	75	592
1982	75	595
1983	74	595
1984	75	587
1985	78	598
1986	78	594
1987	78	585
1988	78	[a]
1989	78	[a]
1990	74	[a]
1991	74	[a]

[a]Centers are no longer funded in terms of beds, but in terms of patient-days.

committee to the GCRC branch (all extramural scientists); these recommendations are forwarded to the Council of the Division of Research Resources (DRR), which is the funding component. The usual award period is 5 years. Since 1970, a number of GCRCs have been discontinued and a few others activated; in 1991, the total number of centers stood at 74.

In contrast to the NIH Clinical Center, which consists of some 12 disease-oriented hospitals, the GCRCs have a *general* research orientation; that is, they serve all departments in their medical schools and are not single-disease or single-discipline oriented. Today's 78 GCRCs vary in bed capacity from 4 to 30, with corresponding variations in staff size. Most of them are designed for the study of adult patients, but nine are pediatric and seven are mixed. There is also one perinatal center for the study of mothers prior to term and their infants at term. Another is exclusively an out-patient center, and still another is a dental research center. The Rockefeller Hospital was awarded GCRC support for the first time in 1963 and has always been the largest in the number of funded beds (30 in 1990); it admits all age groups.

A number of medical schools have more than one GCRC: today's 78 centers are located at 55 medical schools and 3 free-standing biomedical research institutions (Rockefeller, MIT, and Scripps Clinic). Every pediatric center is administered by a school that also has an adult center. Johns Hopkins has four centers (adult, pediatric, aging, and out-patient); Harvard has centers at each of four major teaching hospitals (Beth Israel, Brigham and Women's, Children's, and Massachusetts General); the University of California (San Francisco) has three centers (adult and pediatric at Moffitt General, and adult at the San Francisco General, a county hospital). GCRCs tend to be sited in the most research-intensive medical schools (defined by AAMC as a rank ordering of schools in terms of federal dollars received annually for research), as seen in Fig. 10–2. Thirty-seven schools in the top 40 had GCRCs, 18 schools in the middle 40, and 3 in the bottom 47 schools. From another perspective, 69 of the 127 U.S. medical schools in 1987 had no GCRCs.

The GCRC program has been assigned administratively to the Division of Research Resources since 1969. Thus, the performance of the GCRC branch is overseen by the Council of DRR, and not by any of the Institute Councils, all of which are categorical (that is, disease-oriented); this is consistent with the general, non-categorical intent of the GCRC program. Today's 78 centers vary not only in size and budgetary needs, but also in the kinds of POR performed in each of them; this individuality is considered a strength of the program.

A SURVEY OF THE GCRC PROGRAM IN 1987

In 1987 I gained permission from the GCRC branch to carry out a confidential survey of all 78 GCRCs through their program directors; it was my intention to learn the views of these directors on the past, present, and future of POR at their respective sites. Five program directors chose not to take part in this survey. Thus, the conclusions I have reached are based on information from 73 of the 78 centers.

The process was carried out in two phases. First, a questionnaire was mailed to each program director after he had agreed to participate (via a personal telephone call). The questionnaire was designed to gather simple factual information about staff numbers and duties, along with the director's subjective views on such matters as trends in the quality of research and the strength of the center's support by the several institutional elements of the medical school.

Then, after receipt of the questionnaire, I clarified all uncertainties by telephone, at which time an appointment was made with each director for the second phase of the survey—a prolonged telephone interview (1 to 2 hours in all cases). The purpose of this interview was to become better acquainted with each direc-

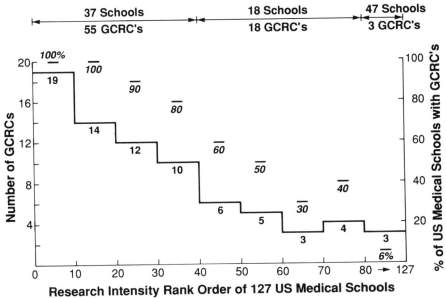

Fig. 10–2   Sitings of 76 GCRCs in 127 U.S. medical schools (1987) in relation to their research-intensity rank order. (GCRC data provided by James F. O'Donnell, GCRC Branch, 1987; research-intensity rank orders from Donna J. Williams, AAMC, Section for Operational Studies, 1988)

tor, and to gather impressions informally about the status of POR in that institution and the nature of POR in that center. This laborious but highly informative exercise was carried out over a 12-month period and completed in 1988.

I would have preferred to copy the Flexner model of 1910 by paying a personal visit to each center, but time and expense precluded such a plan. (I am still awed by Flexner's ability to visit 155 medical schools in less than 12 months, all by train; a pilot study carried out with my travel agent showed that Flexner's performance could not be matched today, even at the speed of air travel!) I am extremely grateful to the 73 program directors who gave generously of their time and cooperation in a venture that most of them enthusiastically supported.

Personnel and Physical Characteristics of 73 GCRCs in 1987

Table 10–2 summarizes some of the factual data obtained by questionnaire from the 73 program directors. Most of these directors held the rank of full professor; 64 centers also employed an associate director, and 16 a second associate director. Most of the program directors were affiliated with departments of medicine, and 43 of 73 also served as heads of divisions. The dominant specialty of these directors was endocrinology (36 of 73 directors).

The salaries of the directors came from several sources in addition to partial support from the GCRC award. Income derived from service to private patients and funneled through their departmental budgets was earned by 48 of 73 direc-

Table 10–2   Survey of 73 General Clinical Research Centers (1987)[a]

1. *Program Directors*
   a. Years of service as PD   Median, 6 (range, 1–27)
   b. Rank: Professor   64
              Assoc. prof.   7
              Asst. prof.   2
              Tenured   65
   c. Departmental affiliation
              Medicine   56
              Pediatrics   12
              Other   5
              Serving also as a division head   43
   d. Primary specialty
              Endocrinology   36
              Hematology   5
              Mineral metabolism   5
              Scattered   27
   e. Salary: multiple sources, with part from GCRC: 70
                            and part from private practice: 48 (via departmental budgets)
   f. Research funding: multiple sources with part from personal grants: 69
   g. PDs as major users of GCRC facilities: 47

2. *Other Staff Members* (salaried wholly or in part by the center)
   a. Assoc. PDs: In 64 centers (and second assoc. PD in 16)
   b. PhDs:
              53 in 36 centers (26 full-time)
              5 profs., 12 assoc. profs., 14 asst. profs., 22 other
              7 in biochemistry, 12 in biostatistics, 8 in nutrition, 5 in endocrinology
   c. Physician's assitants: 2
   d. Nurse practitioners: 38 (in 10 centers)
   e. Research nurses: 689 (in 67 centers, none in 6)
                                       (range, 1–31; median, 10)
   f. Research dietitians: 90 (in 68 centers, none in 5)
                                       (range, 1–5; median, 1)

3. *Core Laboratories*
   a. Budgets: 55 on GCRC budget, 4 from other sources
   b. Technical staff: total FTE's 168 (range, 1–7; median, 3)
   c. Major emphasis of laboratory
              Endocrinology   32
              General   12
              Metabolism   4
              Scattered   11
   d. Supervisors
              Professors   23
              Assoc. prof.   15
              Asst. prof.   10
              Other   11

4. *Biostatistics*
   a. Biostatisticians dedicated to GCRC: 9 full-time, 30 part-time
   b. No statistical advice available in 14 centers
   c. Equipment: CLINFO 53, PROPHET 14; 62 have access to other computer facilities

Table 10–2   (Continued)

5. *Personnel in Training*	
a. Residents	Median no. of 10 per year take some part in GCRC activities in 33 centers
b. Medical students	Median no. of 7 per year take some part in GCRC activities in 48 centers
c. MD-PhD candidates	63 centers are located in 46 institutions that have MD-PhD programs; 28 of the 46 are funded by MSTP[b]
	Total no. of candidates = 1,310, of whom 718 are MSTP candidates
	No MD-PhD candidates take any part in GCRC activities in 37 of 63 sites. At 26 other sites, 1–2 candidates per year work at GCRCs in association with investigators using GCRC facilities

[a]Staff members, core laboratories, and training functions.
[b]The Medical Scientist Training Program of NIGMS.

tors and by 49 of 80 associate directors. Research funding of most of these directors was from personal research grants from various sources. Only 47 of 73 program directors considered themselves to be major users of their GCRC facilities, as did 54 of 80 associate directors.

Thirty-six centers employed at least one PhD. Of 53 PhDs employed in all 73 centers, half were full-time staff members, with a spread of specialties in biostatistics, nutrition, biochemistry, and endocrinology.

Nursing staff made up the largest part of the personnel roster, with 38 nurse-practitioners and 689 research nurses; only six centers employed no nurses at all. Ninety research dietitians worked in 68 centers; five centers had no dietitians. In addition to these GCRC-salaried personnel, a large number of other nurses and dietitians took part in the center studies of the many investigator-users and were salaried by the research grants of those outside investigators. Although not shown in Table 10–2, these part-time assistants totaled 27 physician-assistants, 75 nurse-practitioners, 325 research nurses, and 76 research dietitians. Thus, in addition to a total of 817 ancillary staff members who were full-time GCRC employees, there were 503 ancillary staff members who participated in GCRC activities as assistants in the studies of the outside investigators whose grants paid their salaries.

Core laboratories were available to the GCRC users in 59 centers, 55 of which were financed by GCRC funds. Some 168 technical assistants worked in those 59 laboratories, 38 of whom were supervised by tenured professors.

Biostatistical skills were available in 59 of the 73 centers, with a total of 9 full-time and 30 part-time biostatisticians paid partly by GCRC funds but also by other sources. Computer capability was frequently financed by the GCRC program, which supplied the CLINFO system to 53 centers and the PROPHET system to 14.

Medical students and residents played very minor roles in most GCRC operations on a part-time rotational basis, although a few centers made major efforts to involve students and residents in the daily activities. MD-PhD candidates took almost no part in the GCRCs at their institutions, although MD-PhD training programs existed at 63 of the 73 center sites.

To recapitulate, the special facilities made available by the GCRC program are intended to facilitate high-quality POR through the dedication of in-patient and out-patient facilities and trained personnel. The directors and their staffs (nursing, laboratory, biostatistics, and nutrition) are available to assist colleagues from any of the medical school departments in designing and implementing studies. In GCRCs, special attention can be paid to the timing of observations and the collection of samples for laboratory analysis with a degree of care and finesse that is simply not feasible in general hospital wards and out-patient clinics.

The demand for these special services has changed in recent years; in addition, there have been important trends in research directions. This survey was designed to explore these changes by obtaining certain kinds of information at three time points: 1975, 1980, and 1985.

Time-Trends in GCRC Activities (1975–85)

There has been a major shift from in-patient studies of many days' duration to out-patient procedures performed in a single day. For instance, the median number of out-patient visits in the 73 centers increased from 55,000 per year in 1975 to 151,000 in 1985. The number of PIs utilizing all GCRC facilities rose from a median of 19 in 1975 to 26 in 1985, with the total numbers of PI-users rising from 1,391 to 1,994. During the same period, other physician-scientists working on the teams of PI-users rose from a median of 17 to 26, and from a total number of 1,433 to 2,149. Despite these increases in users, however, there was a 30% decrease in in-patient utilization between 1971 and 1985. Thus, the larger number of users must have been engaged primarily in out-patient studies (1977–87).

The nature of the studies performed in these 73 centers from 1975 to 1985 has not changed a great deal. There has been less concentration on new diseases and new disease phenomena, with none at all in 9 centers in 1975, rising to none in 14 centers in 1985. Pharmacologic studies have increased in number, while attention to specimen-collection has decreased. On the other hand, very little effort is being expended on special patient-needs (such as dialysis, transplantations, and total parenteral nutrition), with none at all in 18 centers in 1975, rising to none in 23 centers in 1985. The claim of the program directors that the largest percentage of GCRC studies was focused on the mechanisms of normal or abnormal physiology—namely, basic POR—is heartening if true.

Subjective Viewpoints of the Program Directors

Without breaking our agreement to hold confidential all survey data and conversations with the 73 program directors, I will now summarize their opinions and views about POR at each of their institutions as of 1987.

1. POR in the institution as a whole seemed to be just keeping pace with current trends, or even to be declining in quality and quantity, according to 52 of 71 responses. But the quality of POR had been improving in the GCRCs themselves (34 of 71 responses), due primarily to better-designed research plans and to an increasing use of new technologies.

2. Institutional support for the GCRC program was strongest among administrators (who consider that the center enhances the prestige of the institution and who welcome the financial assistance of a GCRC award) and among clinical department chairmen and full-time clinical faculty, and weakest among the preclinical departments, residents, and students. However, in almost all cases, institutional support for bench research, especially in the clinical departments, far outweighed that for POR and for the GCRC, possibly because bench research generates a more ample and stable funding base through R01 awards.

Asked whether it would be beneficial for an institution to appoint a dean for research (or someone with a comparable title) charged with responsibility for long-term planning and judicious balancing of priorities in all branches of clinical research, including POR, 25 replied that such a person already existed, 34 favored this action, and 14 disfavored it.

3. Advisory committees to the program directors were considered to be important allies, but 35 of 72 respondents felt that these committees could do a better job reviewing research proposals for scientific merit and ethical issues. Forty-one directors considered their advisory committees to be helpful in strengthening intra-institutional support for their GCRC and in building morale in the GCRC unit (50 responses).

4. Bureaucracies at the institutional level, such as IRBs, and officials dealing with radioactivity clearance, animal experiments, and cost-control offices, were not considered barriers to research by 38–41 of 50 respondents. Although 5–10 respondents complained that these bureaucracies needed streamlining, fewer than 5 found these agencies to be adversarial.

5. High morale and creativity in their GCRC units were considered by 62 of 73 directors to depend on reaching a critical mass of intellectual involvement in their management, activities, and research output; but 44 stated that this mass had not been attained. This was considered to be due to the infrequent meetings of user teams with each other and to the rarity of exchanges of research plans and methods among the various investigators. The size of the enterprise at a given center also was considered an important determinant of critical mass— namely, a minimum of five user-teams operating simultaneously in at least six in-patient research beds or with a minimum of 800 out-patient visits per year.

6. Most PDs considered that training of young investigators in POR required more attention and greater effort at improvement. Apprenticeship with an experienced mentor was considered by 59 of 71 respondents to be the major and most effective training method, but also the one most in need of improvement. Scientific and collegial exchanges among GCRC user teams were considered important in POR training. Thirty-eight directors believed that such exchanges were satisfactory, and 34 urged that they be more strongly promoted. Formal

course work elsewhere in the institution and special POR tutorials were not favored by most of the Directors.

A major stimulus of recruitment to careers in POR is the fellowship opportunity called the "Clinical Associate Program (CAP)," which is available at every center for selection of promising young investigators and their nomination by local authorities. Awards are made in national competition by the Advisory Committee of the GCRC branch and are funded as supplements to a center's GCRC award. Centers may apply for three such appointments in a given 5-year period; awards can run for up to 3 years, with stipends of $42,500 and with $5,000 in research expenses for each appointee. The program directors indicated that they strongly favored this program, and 54 of 73 urged its expansion to enhance recruitment into POR careers and to improve the quantity and quality of POR at their Centers. Yet, the number of clinical associates awarded per year has fallen short of the theoretical maximum (Table 10–3), due in part to lack of funds available to the GCRC branch and in part to weak nomination paperwork.

7. Exposure of medical students and residents to GCRC activities was considered valuable to the GCRC staff, as well as to these temporary participants. At most centers, they were engaged in caring for research patients and taking part in research procedures. Their mentors were mainly the investigators using the centers, not the directors and GCRC staff members. The number of residents

Table 10–3 Clinical Associate Program, GCRC Branch, DRR

Year	No. of New Awards	Total No. in Process	Expenditures on CAP (as % of Total Apportionment to the GCRC Branch)
1974	12	12	
1975	12	13	
1976	6	16	0.9
1977	16	22	1.0
1978	10	30	1.3
1979	18	39	2.1
1980	15	43	2.4
1981	10	45	3.1
1982	20	43	2.5
1983	15	38	2.2
1984	16	48	2.5
1985	18	47	2.6
1986	14	44	2.7
1987	21	39	2.3
1988	10	45	
1989	15	41	
	Average ± S.D. = 42.9 ± 3.3		= 2.5 ± 0.3
Total awards = 228	31 still in process		197 completed

Source: Personal communication, Dr. Bernard Talbot, GCRC Branch, DRR, NIH (May 10, 1990).

taking part in GCRC activities varied greatly, with a median numbers of 7 residents and 7 students. (Ten centers had no contact with students or residents at any time.) The duration of their exposure to the GCRC was not ascertained in this survey; in only half of the centers were there regularly scheduled rotations, and presumably they were brief.

To recapitulate, it is clear that in-patient POR has been decreasing in intensity and that out-patient POR has taken its place. This suggests that utilization of the center as a metabolic ward for long-term studies has been supplanted by studies shortened by the advent of modern technologies, but also by social changes. Fewer patients are willing to be hospitalized for long stays, especially over weekends; and, as patients and spouses, both employed, find that family time is more precious, the attractiveness of hospitalization (even at no expense except time) has greatly decreased.

Program directors are half-salaried (at most) by GRC funds, and must obtain the rest of their salaries from other sources. Thus, program directors have more and more constraints on their time, and many are not major users of their centers. This represents a serious loss of important role models for recruitment of promising young medical graduates into POR careers, a lack that is not adequately compensated for by investigator-users as mentors, for their time is also seriously constrained. The program director who waits for "customers" to request the use of GCRC facilities faces the hazard of increasing under-utilization of that resource. Consequently, he must spend more and more time searching for potential users among those colleagues who have succeeded in winning R01 awards and persuading them to carry out some aspects of their programs in his center.

The impression that GCRCs are simply a convenient resource (like an animal center) rather than an educational center is pervasive. This perception undercuts the recruitment of promising young investigators into POR careers, as does the decrease in the number of effective POR mentors.

The single most important message is that, although GCRCs are elegantly equipped and staffed, their effectiveness is increasingly threatened by time constraints on investigators' workdays. Ways must be found to give these users dedicated time for POR, relieved of many of the duties of teaching and general service to patients that consume so much time and effort.

OTHER SITES FOR POR

It cannot be assumed that POR is performed exclusively in GCRCs: this would overlook the likelihood that certain types of studies can be carried out effectively in intensive-care units, in neonatal nurseries, in specialized disease-oriented centers (cancer, diabetes, genetic disorders, etc.), and even on general wards if tight supervision is unnecessary. Nor is it true that schools without GCRCs are totally unengaged in POR: in fact, of the 164 authors in the 3-D Survey who wrote at least one article identified as Basic POR (Category 1), 17% worked in the 69 U.S. medical schools that had no GCRCs. Nevertheless, there is a strong though imperfect correlation between the performance of POR and an environment enriched by the presence of an active GCRC.

In institutions with GCRCs, it was not possible to assess how much time and effort are devoted to POR *outside* the center. There appeared to be three possible ways to attack this measurement, but preliminary studies showed that none were simple and none were entirely valid. However, a crude approximation to the magnitude of this "other sites" question was attempted by reading a random sample of the 339 Basic POR abstracts in the 3-D Survey (see Table 5–6 for details) for clues to the question of whether GCRC facilities might have been required. To that end, a 20% sample of Basic POR articles in each of the nine cohorts (three departments at three time periods)—i.e., 68 of 339 abstracts—was selected and read for clues to sites of performance. In all three departments, the number of articles reporting studies that might have required GCRC facilities was only one-half to one-third of the total number. If this estimate is generalizable, one-half to two-thirds of the Basic POR at a given institution is being carried out in facilities other than those offered by its GCRC.

THE COST OF POR AT THE CLINICAL CENTER
AND IN THE GCRC PROGRAM

The sums allocated to support POR in the approximately 1,100 beds managed by the Clinical Center and the GCRCs have been falling since 1977 if inflation is taken into account. For instance, in constant (1987) dollars, the total GCRC appropriation has fallen 19% since 1972, although it has remained fairly level since 1984 (Table 10–4); and the total operating budget at the Clinical Center fell 35% from 1977 to 1987 (Table 10–5, line e).

It is now generally accepted that the costs per research patient are better calculated on the basis of "patient-days" than on the number of hospital beds set aside for such patients. The GCRC branch calculates patient-days in terms of the number of in-patient days in a given year spent in a center by all patients whose costs are entirely borne by the center, plus one-third of the number of out-patient visits that year. (As seen in Table 10–5, the Clinical Center makes this calculation somewhat differently, so that strict comparisons of POR costs in these two major sites must be handled with care.)

The patient-day costs of the various GCRCs range widely, due to geographical cost differences as well as to the differing efficiencies of small and large centers. Figure 10–3 shows a bell-shaped curve of costs for 63 of the centers in FY1986, ranging from $125 to $750 per patient-day, with a mode of $450. (The considerably higher costs at 12 centers presumably attracted the attention of managers at the GCRC branch!) In that same year, 1986, the Clinical Center's

Table 10–4 Changes in Cost of the GCRC Program (1960–89)

| Fiscal Year | Apportionment from DRR | |
| | Current Dollars | Constant Dollars (1987 base)[a] |
	(in Thousands)	
1960	3,000	13,656
1961	8,000	35,647
1962	27,000	117,613
1963	33,500	142,057
1964	27,100	112,465
1965	26,900	108,404
1966	28,500	110,836
1967	28,500	106,204
1968	30,400	108,149
1969	35,004	118,195
1970	35,004	111,217
1971	38,004	114,128
1972	42,181	120,161
1973	41,300	112,760
1974	42,320	108,632
1975	42,619	98,831
1976	42,533	91,786
1977	47,283	94,505
1978	51,946	96,671
1979	51,941	89,314
1980	56,720	88,851
1981	60,148	85,333
1982	64,384	84,099
1983	74,520	91,637
1984	81,262	94,332
1985	87,878	96,584
1986	86,554	91,132
1987	92,497	92,497
1988	103,000	97,884
1989	109,000	97,793

[a]According to the Biomedical R&D Price Index, Division of Planning and Evaluation, Office of the NIH Director (December 12, 1988).

cost per patient-day was $1,156. Table 10–5 demonstrates the formulation of Clinical Center costs and the changes in costs from 1977 to 1987.

Total direct costs for all personnel employed in the GCRC program, in constant dollars, did not vary from 1975 to 1987 (data not shown), even though salaries were constantly rising. This was due to a reduction in the number of centers from 84 to 78 and to a reduction in the number of personnel in all categories: professional, administrative, laboratory, dietary, and nursing. At the Clinical Center, on the other hand, the patient-day costs rose from 1977 to 1987 as the number of admissions fell. It is evident that major hospital expenses (like those of large hotels) cannot be reduced simply by admitting fewer patients (or patrons).

Table 10–5 NIH Clinical Center Costs[a] (in 1987 Dollars)

	FY1977	FY1982	FY1987
Basic Data			
a. Total no. of available beds	524	505	490
b. Total no. of hospital days (admission to discharge)	129,680	112,250	106,840
c. Total no. of pass-patient days[b]	11,600	10,000	16,000
d. Total no. of out-patient visits	50,722	48,331	66,680
e. Total CC operating budget			
Millions, current dollars	$96	$110	$125
Millions, 1987 dollars	$192	$168	$125
Calculated Data			
f. Occupancy rate			
(b/365a)	68%	61%	60%
g. Operating costs per bed per day			
(e/365a) (current dollars)	$502	$595	$699
h. Total no. of patient-days[c]			
(b - c) + 0.1d	123,152	107,083	97,508
i. Operating costs per patient-day[c]			
(e/h) (current dollars)	$780	$1,027	$1,282

[a]Exclusive of costs for utilities and maintenance.

[b]Patients "on pass" from the Clinical Center (mainly weekends).

[c]Note that patient-day costs are calculated differently for the 78 GCRCs by the GCRC Branch.

Source: Calculations based on data provided by the Clinical Center Director's Office (Gerald C. Macks, management analyst).

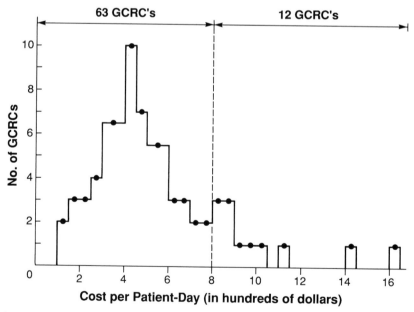

Fig. 10–3 Distribution of costs per patient-day in 75 GCRCs in 1986. (GCRC data provided by Dr. James F. O'Donnell, GCRC Branch, 1988)

STRENGTHS AND WEAKNESSES OF POR OF THE CLINICAL CENTER AND IN THE GCRC PROGRAM

The two major sites of POR in the United States—namely, the NIH Clinical Center and the 74 GCRCs located in many of the leading biomedical institutions throughout the United States—share many (but not all) of the same strengths and weaknesses.

Strengths

1. The most important asset of both organizations is the facility itself—the location isolated from other distracting elements of the host institution and staffed by specially trained nurses, dietitians, and other ancillary personnel. It is a place in which patients (or volunteers) can be studied carefully and quietly, with none of the constraints on hospital stay imposed by cost considerations on non-research patients, for there are no hospital charges and no doctors' fees at these sites.

The average hospital stay in the GCRC system as a whole decreased from 16 days in the 1970s to 4–6 days in 1990; that in the Clinical Center fell from 15 days in 1982 to 12 in 1988. This is due in part to the difficulty of recruiting research patients for hospital stays, especially over weekends, but, more importantly, to the fact that the nature of the research performed on the GCRCs has changed in ways that demand shorter hospital stays. Evidently, long-term balance studies, with total collections of urine and feces and with strict dietary controls, are no longer the mode of study that was standard only 15 years ago. And as patient stays have decreased, more and more studies are being performed on ambulatory patients in out-patient facilities. In Bethesda and elsewhere, these facilities enjoy the same advantages of special staffing and meticulous attention to detail that are characteristic of the in-patient facilities.

2. The relationships between medical staffs and patients are more personal in a POR setting, and the atmosphere is more cooperative, friendly, and cheerful than it is in a busy general hospital ward setting. It is a major asset of GCRCs that patients and staffs see themselves as partners in a cooperative enterprise. This atmosphere of partnership is due largely to the careful selection of appropriate patients for a given study and to the time spent explaining to them the details of a given study, its rationale and safety, and all possible alternatives.

3. Scientifically, the most important asset of a POR facility is the golden opportunity it provides for medical investigators and their staffs to watch carefully and to think deeply about the medical challenges posed by their patients; this forces them to formulate new hypotheses and to devise new stratagems for attacking unsolved questions. There is time to ponder an unexpected event—an unexplained turn in the course of the disease or a puzzling response to a medication—and thus to obtain fresh insights into a disease or a manipulation under study.

4. Another major asset is the proximity of POR facilities to the laboratories of the physician-scientists who have planned the special procedures most relevant to the conditions under study and the manipulations imposed (such as special diets, new drugs, and changes in environmental conditions). Ideally, the physician-investigators are themselves the laboratory investigators; senior investigators who delegate these responsibilities to younger staff members run the risk of overlooking something new and of trivializing their essential role as mentors.

5. A final major advantage enjoyed by GCRC-users is their proximity to the laboratories of scientists who are *not* engaged in POR, but whose experience and skills can be called on in devising new procedures and in applying new technologies not yet familiar to the GCRC users themselves. Non-POR scientists with skills in physics, chemistry, mathematics, biochemistry, molecular biology, or behavioral science have interestingly different viewpoints about human health and disease that can be stimulating and provocative for those physician-scientists who may see problems more narrowly and from a strictly medical viewpoint.

Regrettably, there are many biomedical scientists who, lacking familiarity with POR, believe that POR facilities exist simply to act as the final step in translating the flashes of genius of laboratory scientists into clinical reality. Indeed, Simon Flexner, the first director of the Rockefeller Institute, was committed to this proposition and conceived of the Rockefeller Hospital as a test site for the bright ideas generated in the Institute's laboratories. In fact, this has happened only rarely. During my 40 years at the Rockefeller Hospital, I recall only one instance in which a laboratory observation by biochemists was turned into a testable hypothesis in patients—namely, the treatment of sickle-cell crises with cyanate.

Indeed, the traffic of ideas often runs the other way, from clinical observations to explorations at the laboratory level. One thinks of the demonstration that sickle-cell hemoglobin differs in molecular structure from ordinary hemoglobin. That remarkable discovery originated in a clinician's vivid description to a physical chemist of his quandry over the episodic nature of the sickling of red cells among victims of that disease (from W.B. Castle, the clinician, to Linus Pauling, the chemist, as described by Strauss, 1964).

Whether one traffic pattern of ideas dominates over another between bench and bedside is irrelevant; what really matters is that this two-way bridge be kept open at all times (and toll-free).

Difficulties and Weaknesses

1. POR is the most difficult type of biomedical research because of the many biologial and psychological variables that are difficult or impossible to control. Nevertheless, the existence of multiple variables is a characteristic of any whole organism, be it man or other species. If we are to succeed in gaining a better understanding of any whole organism, we must learn to accept the variables—to minimize some, eliminate others, and work with the rest.

2. Studies in man are expensive in comparison to bench research. The

GCRC award pays for the medical and nursing care, special diets, drugs, and routine laboratory expenses of patients admitted for research studies; these costs amount (in the average GCRC) to some $500 per patient-day. But research patients also deserve and get the best medical care, and when costly diagnostic or experimental procedures are indicated, these costs must be passed along to third-party payers (when this is possible) or covered by the research grants of the investigator teams that use GCRCs for their studies. At the Clinical Center, all costs for an Institute's research patients are paid out of the Institute's intramural research funds. These costs are being met more and more grudgingly by the Institutes' directors, because many who control the budget think that such funds are better spent on the bench research of non-clinical researchers.

3. The salary of a bedside researcher at the Clinical Center is assured so long as the position exists, while in U.S. medical schools the salaries of most researchers are derived from "soft" monies—largely from externally funded grants such as R01 awards. In the case of the GCRC program director, only half of his salary can come from the GCRC award; the rest must be made up out of other grant funds or by caring for private patients, or both. (Service to patients generates income for department budgets, which in turn pays back some of it in the form of an institutional salary.) Currently, the GCRC branch requires program directors to be PIs on one or more R01 grants (or comparable peer-reviewed support from some other source); with today's 30% or lower award rates for R01s, this rule imposes one more heavy burden on the program director's time and energy.

Bedside scientists at the Clinical Center do not compete for grants, as do the GCRC investigators; but at the NIH, there is strong competition for funds by the non-clinical scientists whose laboratory expenses come out of the same pocket as monies spent on bedside research. Thus, both sets of POR workers have major budgetary problems; they are simply different in origin and kind.

4. Strong institutional support is the keystone of success in almost every human endeavor. At the Clinical Center, 12 separate Institutes support POR, with differing degrees of enthusiasm; for the 78 GCRCs, some enjoy strong institutional support, others do not. The support for POR by deans and department chairmen (on the one hand) and by scientific directors of the 12 Institutes (on the other) is continually competed for by demands made by the many other components under their control. For instance, in medical schools, there are conflicting interests among a host of pre-clinical and clinical departments; the difficult balance of the competing costs of education, service, and research; the pressure of community interests; and the cost and complexity of regulation by government. And at the NIH, there exists a delicate balance between scientific objectives and congressional imperatives—the conviction that the prestige of an Institute depends more on its basic science than on its clinical accomplishments, and thus the tendency to allocate intramural research funds to laboratory science rather than to bedside research.

In 1987 the President's Office of Management and Budget requested an in-depth analysis of the NIH intramural operation, testing the proposition that privatization of the NIH would produce a better product at less expense. An IOM committee chaired by Harold T. Shapiro carried out this review and concluded in 1988 that privatization of the NIH was highly undesirable, and that, indeed, the NIH intramural process was healthy. However, among many plaudits there crept in the recognition that the scientific directors of the various Institutes enjoyed powerful control over both the science and the budgets of their Institutes, but with minimal accountability. The committee strongly recommended a vigorous and periodic process of external review of all intramural operations (IOM Report, 1988a, p. 8). In response, the NIH director called together an external consultant panel chaired by Robert L. Hill to review this and other recommendations. The Hill committee's 1990 reply urged that "the scientific and administrative performance of [all] scientific directors should be evaluated every 4 years by the boards of scientific counselors" and that the process itself be re-evaluated every 2 years by a panel consultant to the NIH Director (see NIH Advisory Committee, 1990, p. 29). These recommendations were not received happily by the scientific directors, and it is too early to judge their usefulness.

5. The size and complexity of operations at NIH and at U.S. medical schools diminish the collegiality that was once maintained at smaller work sites. The dominance today of reductionism over integrative science has created a two-culture gap that varies in width and depth with the size of the institution. Because the NIH is so large and its staffs are so dispersed, the two-culture problem may have more serious implications there than in U.S. medical schools. It is the obligation of leadership to ameliorate this problem; wherever leadership is not strongly supportive, the morale of POR investigators at almost all sites has fallen to low levels.

6. Recruitment of young MDs into research of any kind has become increasingly difficult in the last 20 years, and for POR the recruitment problem is more marked than for other categories of clinical research. There are many reasons: the weakness of institutional support for POR in comparison to bench research, the lengthening odds against winning R01 funding for POR, and the insecurity of research careers that depend on outside funding, to name a few. Even at the NIH, the glamour of spending a few years at NIH training as an MD research associate has faded in comparison to those years of the doctor draft during the Korean and Vietnam wars when service at the NIH attracted superb candidates nationwide. Recruitment of the best young MDs to the NIH has now become a vexing problem.

7. Training for bench research is clearly route-marked. And with the inauguration of FIRST awards, K11 awards, and the Medical Scientist Training Program (MSTP), the funds for such training have kept pace with the demand. For aspiring reductionists, the road is clearly marked but long. In contrast, there is no comparable training pathway for MDs who choose to pursue a career in POR and no agreed-upon best method for that training. Nor are there funds specifically earmarked for this purpose.

The blame for this situation must be laid at the door of senior POR researchers themselves. Unlike those biochemists and molecular biologists who have initiated and dominated most MD-PhD programs, clinical researchers have been slow to recognize the need for advanced training of MDs for research careers, slow in devising such programs, and slow in securing funding for them. There are a few notable exceptions: for instance, a small but well-organized training program at Pittsburgh University under the Department of Medicine, and another at a small number of pediatric centers under the leadership of the Association of Medical School Pediatric Department Chairmen; a small but vigorous program in research cardiology run by the Sarnoff Foundation, and one in nutrition funded by the Pew Charitable Trusts.

While the needs far exceed the means, neither will be met unless the leaders in POR define their training goals more clearly, then create new opportunities and take advantage of them. This is nowhere better illustrated than in their halting embrace of the CAP program organized by the GCRC branch in 1975. If, as some would argue, the only road to survival for any sort of clinical researcher is the attainment of a double degree (MD-PhD), then POR mentors must seek a way to intrude on the turf of their local MSTP (or other MD-PhD program) and win places for POR-minded applicants in this society of highly selected, tuition-free students.

8. Bureaucratic barriers to POR are widely perceived to cause serious delays in exploring new investigative ideas, and of these, the usual target is the IRB that monitors research on human beings at every U.S. research institution. According to federal law, an IRB must be informed of all research plans that involve human subjects. The plans must be described fully, and guarantees must be demonstrated that will protect the safety and confidentiality of the research subject. The board's approval must be obtained before applications for funding can be awarded by the NIH, and this approval process can take several months. (The NIH has a similar review process supervised by the director of the Clinical Center.)

The quality and efficiency of IRB review seem to vary greatly from one institution to another. It is regrettable that this review conforms to no standardized format and that there is no formal accreditation process on a national level for this process. No one disputes the need for and worth of such protective measures; the fact that such protection can be assured expeditiously in some institutions but not in others indicates that the perceived "barrier" is not inherent in the objectives but in the manner in which certain boards operate. Similar reviews must be carried out to certify the safe and humane use of animals in experimental studies, as well as all uses of radioactive isotopic materials. All are completely justified assurances and can be managed speedily if the relevant panels are well organized.

The perception of bureaucratic barriers to POR is widely held, but it is groundless and seems to have stemmed from the fact that these safeguards did not exist 20 years ago but do now. They are in fact a protection to investigators as well as to patients acting as research subjects.

9. A major weakness of POR at all sites is the threat to innovativeness that stems from thinking in terms of minutely detailed protocols of all research plans,

an operational mode that has been promoted by the practices and predilections of IRBs and DRG study sections. For certain kinds of clinical research, a strict protocol is an absolute necessity. In large controlled trials of new drugs or new procedures, and even in small trials testing drug safety, certain rigidly prescribed observations must be carried out at predetermined intervals. But the essence of innovative research is the exploration of an idea, the outcome of which the investigator cannot predict. To demand that such explorations be described in advance, with descriptions of what is to be examined and exactly when, is to substitute ritual for inquisitiveness. Protocol-mindedness inhibits an investigator from looking for unexpected developments that might lead him in a different direction. If working in an atmosphere of uncertainty is indeed the hallmark of innovative research, then adherence to a rigid protocol is its antithesis.

Exploratory research (looking for leads) must be promoted by every means. Only when these leads have clearly revealed the best pathway has the time arrived for drawing up strict guidelines with which to obtain clear proof of the validity of a hypothesis. Step 1 is the "fishing expedition," a term that, sadly, has fallen into disrepute as investigators, hedging their bets and playing it safe, fall back on increasingly certain means and goals. Protocol-mindedness and short-term objectives have replaced long-term programs and broad themes of research, to the detriment of innovation.

10. Scientific review of ongoing POR by knowledgeable outsiders is by no means the rule at all POR sites. The GCRC program guarantees this kind of review only every 5 years, when individual grants come up for competitive renewal. At renewal time, a project-site visit is arranged; this entails bringing some 15 outside experts to the site in question, to hear six or eight major users of that center describe what they have done and plan to do in the future—all in about 20 minutes per investigator, with about 10 minutes for questions from the visitors. The best feature of this process (and its rehearsals prior to the visit) is that the major users hear about each other's progress and future plans, often for the first time. It is the rare center that regularly schedules meetings of its users to discuss ongoing research studies more than once every 5 years.

The infrequency of internal reviews of research programs in many GCRCs is a serious weakness; but none of the GCRCs, to my knowledge, have arranged for systematic annual reviews by outsiders. This deficiency is even more striking at the NIH. The only extramural review of clinical programs of research within each Institute at NIH is one that is performed every 3 or 4 years by its Board of Scientific Counselors. This board is far more concerned with its Institute's nonclinical laboratory research than with its bedside research. Indeed, board members are usually selected by a scientific director on the basis of their competence in a given research area of laboratory research; the boards' reviews of POR at the Clinical Center are rarely more than superficial.

In 1985, the first (and only) NIH Clinical Center Review was carried out under the chairmanship of Donald W. Seldin; his committee reviewed all aspects of the Clinical Center—administrative, financial, and scientific. One subcommittee of eight members reviewed 50 research protocols, chosen for review by the director of the Clinical Center on the basis of their heavy usage of the center's facilities and as representatives of high-quality research. "There was substantial variation in the quality of the protocols reviewed, from truly outstanding to quite poor, and there was also considerable variation in quality in and among the Institutes. *Reviewers agreed that some proposals would not pass the scrutiny of the extramural peer review process*" (p. 44) [emphasis mine].

In 1988 the Shapiro committee set up by IOM to review the NIH intramural system made no mention at all of the quality of bedside research being pursued in the Clinical Center. Nor in 1990 did an Advisory Committee to the NIH director responding to the Shapiro report make any comment on the quality of POR in the Clinical Center, nor whether the research opportunities under the surveillance of the Clinical directors of the 12 Institutes were being properly utilized.

If, indeed, the quality of POR has declined in recent decades, as many critics have complained, then nothing could be more salutary than initiation of a review process carried out by outside experts at every GCRC and in the clinical operation of every NIH Institute. Advisory committees could serve three very useful functions: (1) their review of ongoing research will be provocative as well as helpful; (2) they will share with the leadership of a given POR site the difficult decisions on whether certain researchers deserve continued support and others do not; and (3) their growing attachment to and interest in a given center will lift the morale of the entire staff of that center.

SUMMARY AND CONCLUSIONS

POR has been carried out in sites specially equipped for that activity for only the last 80 years, with an impressive expansion of these special facilities starting in the 1950s. At present, the major dedicated sites for POR are the 500-bed NIH Clinical Center and the 74 GCRCs throughout the United States. In addition, some types of POR are performed at other locations in U.S. medical centers, such as intensive care unites, neonatal centers, cancer centers, and even the general wards, but the quantity of POR carried on in these non-dedicated places has not been measured. The total cost of operating the two major POR programs (the Clinical Center and the GCRCs) amounts to about $300 million per year, or about 4% of the total NIH appropriation.

To measure the *quality* of POR studies and the enthusiasm with which they are supported locally, I initiated a detailed review of 73 GCRC programs by lengthy questionnaires and telephone conversations with their program directors, and by personal interviews with the 12 clinical directors at the (then) 12 Institutes that used the facilities of the Clinical Center. To sum up my impressions in a single sentence, I concluded that POR at both major sites is being performed with greater difficulty and with weaker institutional support than ever before.

There are enough exceptions to this statement to prove that this enterprise *can* succeed, brilliantly, especially if it is reinvigorated with new ideas and stronger leadership.

The strengths and weaknesses of the two major POR sites are described in detail. The strengths are numerous and powerful, the weaknesses remediable. If at individual locations the weaknesses do not yield to critical self-examination, accountability for the considerable cost of POR in this country can be obtained only by a vigorous system of external review performed at regular intervals by rotating panels of extramural experts in POR.

11

Training MDs for Biomedical Research

John Gardner, in his searching essays on leadership (1990), quotes an old French axiom: "Be sure you want the consequences of what you want." The wisdom of this adage is rarely heeded. Leaders in many walks of life decide what they want and persuade their constituents to follow their lead, but all too often, they fail to look ahead to the consequences of getting what they so earnestly wanted and won. Perhaps the most timely example of this un-wisdom is the failure, 45 years after Hiroshima, to have faced up to the manifold problems of radioactive waste disposal.

Indeed, Gardner's French maxim would not be a bad choice to adorn the portals of the U.S. Congress, or to serve as a postscript to its opening prayers. Equally appropriately, it could serve as an addendum to the Hippocratic Oath, reminding physicians and medical scientists that much more is involved in medical progress than simply keeping more people alive longer.

From the beginning of the modern era of the NIH under C. J. Van Slyke's reorganization, training was an equal partner with the pursuit of scientific progress in promoting the health of the U.S. population. Over the next 40 years, many training programs were launched by NIH (and a few abandoned) aimed at meeting the training needs of its many constituents—pre-doctoral and post-doctoral applicants, MDs, PhDs, and other degree holders; minorities and women; senior investigators in mid-career; and promising newcomers. The total cost of these many training programs has run into the billions of dollars; the Medical Scientist Training Program (MSTP) alone has invested more than $400 million in some 2,000 double-degree graduates since it began in 1960. Can we be sure that these efforts have been worthwhile?

To respond to that question with more than simple faith in the answer forces us to attempt to measure the consequences of providing what we felt was so obviously wanted—namely, more biomedical scientists who were better equipped by their training to become productive and independent investigators. But such accounting has rarely been satisfying. Indeed, a 1988 IOM Committee Report, "Resources for Clinical Investigation," called loudly for "data to document the record of training programs in producing effective clinical investigators."

Perhaps the major difficulty in setting up such an accounting has been the word "effective." Aside from the distinctions that must be made between high-quality innovative research and research that simply meets high standards of performance, what are the criteria for success in evaluating training programs designed to produce researchers who have high standards and may or may not be outstandingly innovative?

In recent years, several noteworthy attempts have been made to measure the effectiveness of the training programs financed by NIH and by agencies in the private sector. A groundbreaker was the 1983 Rand Corporation report, "The Supply of Physician Researchers," undertaken for the Hartford Foundation by Carter et al.; then the 1986 IOM-NAS Committee Report, "The Career Achievements of NIH Postdoctoral Trainees and Fellows," by Garrison and Brown; and finally, a second Rand Corporation report for the NIH in 1987, "An Evaluation of the NIH Research Career Development Award," by Carter et al. In all cases, the "success" of training was measured in terms of three types of individual achievement: the ability of awardees to obtain research funding after completion of their training, their subsequent employment record as an index of career progress, and the number and citation counts of their research publications. By all these measures MDs and PhDs who had been awarded training grants were more "successful" than those who had applied for but not won such awards.

Whether the training experience itself was responsible for producing more successful scientists could not be concluded. It could be argued that the outcome was predetermined by the selection process. In other words, selectees who were educated in the most prestigious graduate schools, spent their training years in the most research-intensive institutions, and were subsequently employed in such institutions tended to do better than the groups with which they were compared. This unsurprising conclusion fails to distinguish whether these successes were due to training per se or to the criteria for selection of the most likely winners. It can validly be argued that bright, hard-working, highly motivated, and curious young people, if supported financially for several training years and protected from the distractions of responsibilities other than the performance of their research, will do more research, publish more papers, remain better funded, and earn promotions more quickly than others not thus supported.

The question "how many biomedical scientists must be trained to meet the demands for such scientists in the coming years?" remains unanswered today, even after nine mandated reports by the National Research Council (NRC) to Congress since 1974. The ninth NRC-IOM Report on Personnel Needs, "Biomedical and Behavioral Research Scientists: Their Training and Supply" (1989) (chairman, Gerald S. Levey) finally abandoned the formal demand-and-supply projection models previously used, because the data on careers of physician-scientists were judged to be uninterpretable. The number most commonly bandied about is 1,000 new recruits each year (Burns, 1984; Nathan, 1987), but the logic of that guesstimate is far from convincing.

This chapter examines the training needs of medical graduates entering careers in biomedical research, describes the opportunities that currently exist for obtaining this training, and considers the means used to persuade newly graduated MDs to consider careers in research. The following chapter examines the pros and cons of enlisting PhDs in clinical departments and defends the conclu-sion that, with new and improved partnerships between MDs and PhDs, we have the best possible means of addressing the unsolved medical problems facing the public today and tomorrow.

THE NEED FOR MORE SCIENTIFIC TRAINING OF MDs

Changes in medical education after World War II at both the under-graduate and post-graduate levels have led to a succession of graduating classes whose mem-bers Bishop (1984) called "scientific illiterates." Even as long ago as 1971, Eichna called the modern medical school curriculum "overstuffed"—packed with an ever-increasing number of facts that must be memorized in order to pass a succession of competency tests during the medical school years and later (li-censing examinations, specialty and subspecialty boards). With medical science becoming increasingly complex and with time finite, laboratory courses have been shortened or eliminated. Free time in which to explore in the medical li-braries or to become better acquainted with the teaching staff is almost unheard of. Since excellence in teaching is now less esteemed and less well rewarded than research productivity, teachers interact with students less often and less personally. Medical graduates become walking encyclopedias of up-to-date, practical medical knowledge, and their residency years and subspecialty training experiences equip them to be extremely competent practitioners; but any fire of curiosity is likely to have been damped down by the overriding necessity to acquire the facts and figures needed to pass the next test.

No wonder then that, since 1962, when Kunkel bemoaned the lack of training of MDs in the science of medicine and chided the investigator elite for failing to provide such experience, there has been a torrent of essays, speeches, and edi-torials predicting that, if MDs failed to acquire training in biochemistry (later, cell biology, immunology, and, most recently, molecular biology), clinical in-vestigation would become the exclusive province of PhDs and MD-PhDs. Daughaday (1970) pointed out the training opportunities that can exist in sub-specialty fellowships, but Kipnis (1979, 1983) noted how rarely that training is anything more than the acquisition of procedural clinical skills.

By way of remedy, Goldstein (1986) and Carpenter (1988) demanded that MDs undertake several years of additional training in pre-clinical laboratory set-tings in time "protected" from clinical duties (Kelley, 1984). Levey et al. (1981) described a 2-year course in modern laboratory techniques offered to medical department residents and taught exclusively by PhDs. Glickman (1985) pointed to the 5-year training experience in bench research that Physician Scientist Awards (K11 and K12) make available to MDs after 2–3 years of residency training.

It is evident from this small sampling of viewpoints on the need for further scientific training of MDs that medical schools do not now offer the kind and amount of exposure to the scientific aspects of medicine that can qualify their graduates for careers in biomedical research in competition with PhDs and MD-PhDs. Indeed, most new MDs are perfectly content with this situation. They traditionally aim to become competent medical practitioners, and they usually achieve this goal. But fewer and fewer of them are equipped to cope with today's research technologies, to know how to ask good scientific questions, and to capitalize on the opportunities for medical progress that are presented to them by the illnesses of their patients. And at the Establishment level, it is not at all clear how many inquiring minds are needed to keep the research enterprise alive and well.

Surely, if more such people are needed, then the reforms in medical education that are required must be sought at many levels—during the college years, at medical school, and in the postgraduate years of house-staff experience and specialty training. Reforms of such magnitude can only be undertaken by means of a radical shakeup and restructuring of these three educational components, each of which now operates independently of the others. This re-structuring, though fundamental to the future prosperity of both medical education and clinical research, is a matter of such magnitude that it falls outside the limits of this book; fortunately, a few others are engaged with it. Until that day arrives, the young MDs who are research-minded (only a small minority of each school's graduating class) must put up with the hard fact that most of the training opportunities for careers in research begin to apply only after completion of the residency. (MD-PhD programs are the exception, and they will be considered as a special case.)

A CONSIDERABLE DIGRESSION ON GENERALITIES

Given a young medical school graduate who is not satisfied that what he has learned thus far is the Last Word, the preceptors who are intrigued with his curiosity and eager to lure him into a research career would advise the following course of training aimed at achieving the status of independent physician-scientist-investigator. First, spend 2–3 years in house-staff residencies in order to acquire the confidence that comes from having full personal responsibility for patients' welfare. This experience should be followed by no less than 2 years on a training grant in one of the clinical subspecialties, learning the special skills and exposures to clinical disease of that specialty, but (and this is the key advice) attached to a research-minded mentor who is sincerely interested in the intellectual growth of his trainee. If the trainee learns that he is capable of going further in research, he then applies for a fellowship that will allow him much more time for research, free of most of the distractions of departmental and divisional duties and day-to-day clinical responsibilities. No longer a trainee but a Fellow (for at least 2 years), he will address an important but modest clinical research problem, again under the supervision of interested mentors. This experience will put him in a position to apply for funding as an independent researcher—indeed, for R01 funding. In a world more ideal than today's, he will stand an even chance of winning an R01 award, and will then be off and running (at the age of about 32!).

This scenario depicts a progression that Gasser would have approved in 1951: train the putative researcher in the *meaning* of research—its style and historical background—and build on his eagerness to tackle a problem with probes that successfully explore the hypothesis (and probably a succession of hypotheses before finding the right one). The lesson is: ensure that this trained person becomes capable of recognizing new research opportunities and knows how to capitalize on them. Contra today's mode, make it possible for the young person to become truly research-minded first, on the assumption that productive research careers are guaranteed to those with well-prepared minds. *In still other words, support people, not projects.*

The success of this approach, however removed it may be from today's realities, depends on experienced mentors—their presence, their availability, and their willingness to act like mentors. But it also depends on institutional factors: physical as well as intellectual resources for teaching and research, and dedication to the development of an exceptional faculty. Institutions must be devoted to more than the advancement of institutional prestige: the acclaim of rival schools through research "firsts" and other public relations plaudits, the garnishing of patents and of indirect costs from research grants, and bowing to community demands. And, of course, it depends importantly on the candidates themselves—their ability to evaluate their own career objectives and to measure the strength of institutional dedication to research training, especially as it is expressed in terms of protected time (Applegate and Williams, 1990).

What we have today is, in fact, a bewildering complex of conflicting interests that impede the selection of the best candidates for further training. On the national level, we see major differences in support by the private and public sectors: foundations more interested in the development of people as researchers, and industry increasingly dependent on the output of academe but tilted toward the applications of research that will justify devoting funds to training. Even in the NIH, the behemoth of training programs, there is a basic conflict between the mission orientation of the several Institutes and the project orientation of the DRG study sections—the first seemingly more focused on the development of people, the second on research results. And among the several Institutes, a wide spectrum of priorities that each Institute sets up for the funding of training leads to twofold differences in their training paylines.

At the local level, there are the time-dishonored conflicts between MDs and PhDs that are reflected in the different hiring preferences of the pre-clinical and clinical departments. The pre-clinical group, much more dependent than the second on tuition income, has first crack at the incoming medical school classes and can select from each year's harvest the few who show special curiosity and ability. The result: many of these bright young apprentices will remain tied to bench research after graduation. The clinical groups, increasingly dependent on income generated by service to patients, attract those students with a primary interest in human disease, most of whom intend to practice medicine in one or another subspecialty. And, at the institutional level, there are concerns about local fund-raising from donors who can be appealed to on behalf of young aspiring scientists, but also for national acclaim that is reflected in the institution's drawing power for the best medical students, residents, and faculty. The result: a confusing mixture of training programs blown by many winds—philosophical goals but also local and national interests. It is no wonder that the "ideal" is rarely realized.

Unfortunately, there is no compendium of information on training grants offered by the private sector. The 1983 Rand report noted that as many as 75 research foundations support training programs for MDs and PhDs, but that estimate is long out of date. And there appears to be no listing of training mechanisms offered specifically by industry. The Rand study reported that in 1981 private foundations funded about 400 individual early faculty and post-doctoral awards to MDs. In the same year, the NIH awarded about 2,000 training and fellowship awards to MDs and about 3,400 to PhDs (NIH Databook, 1989, Table 39).

Despite its smaller size, private sector support is more important than its numbers suggest. It is highly selective and people-oriented, and it deserves to be more widely known to potential applicants. With no comprehensive listing of support mechanisms by U.S. private foundations, it is not known today whether those offerings have increased or decreased since 1981.

Lacking private sector data, we are driven to focus on the opportunities offered by NIH today—what they are, for whom, by whom judged, and their trends over time. These programs do not follow the logic described in the digression above; they are a patchwork of grants that have proliferated in response to different challenges perceived at various times. The following catalogue will note the key decision makers who select the winners for each program, and whether a program focuses on the development of individuals as researchers or on the production of research results. However the effectiveness of these training programs is measured, at this point it can be said with confidence that the single most important justification for each program is the *protected time* it offers in which individual awardees can grow wiser and acquire research skills, funded by enough dollars to ensure intellectual development without distractions by other responsibilities.

PhD post-doctoral students are not encumbered by these other responsibilities under most circumstances, so MDs are peculiarly benefited by receiving training and fellowship awards. Nevertheless, in 1987, 46% of the post-doctoral trainee awards and 80% of the fellowship awards went to PhDs. The reasons for this imbalance are quite apparent: there are more PhDs graduating in the life sciences each year than MD graduates. MDs train longer in medicine and have larger educational debts to repay, and thus are delayed by several years in initiating their research training. In addition, MDs appointed to positions in clinical departments are expected to help generate their own salaries by providing service to patients.

CLINICAL RESEARCH TRAINING AND CAREER DEVELOPMENT OPPORTUNITIES

Consider the broad array of training and career development opportunities offered by the NIH to anyone planning a career in clinical research—to prospective medical students, MDs or PhDs. Figure 11–1 plots these programs along a time axis symbolic of a student's progress to and through medical school, and during the critically important transition period between house-staff experience and full independence as the PI of a Traditional Research Project award (R01 grant). (Because it is a special case, the MSTP will be discussed separately after the other programs are described).

The array of training experiences that faces a recently graduated MD poses a number of key questions: What kind of research does that graduate hope to perform when he finally attains a position as a full-time assistant professor in a clinical or pre-clinical department? What kind of training award most appropriately fits that objective? What are the chances of success in winning one or another type of training award? Can the applicant survive on the stipend offered while managing to defer re-payment of considerable educational expenses? What facilities and mentorship can a given institution provide during the tenure of whatever award is finally won? Is the institution prepared to offer protected time to its trainees and fellows?

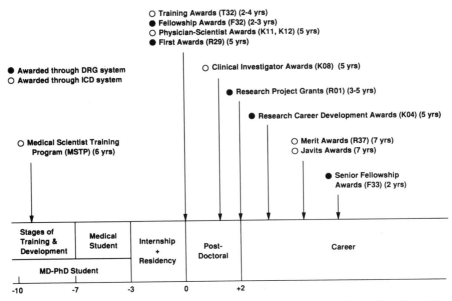

Fig. 11–1   Research training and career development opportunities offered by NIH (1980).

TRAINING GRANTS AND FELLOWSHIP AWARDS

Post-doctoral training grants (T32) for MDs and PhDs are offered by the several NIH Institutes to U.S. medical schools and research institutions on a competitive basis, with renewal applications after 5 years. T32 awards vary in size and cost from one recipient institution to another, depending on their training objectives and capabilities; the selection of post-doctoral awardees is delegated entirely to the training grant directors in those institutions. A given institution may be the recipient of several T32 awards, each training in a different research area or clinical subspecialty.

For MDs, the T32 award formerly made available a year or more of training in one of the subspecialties of medicine, but because this time in training was more often directed at acquiring clinical competence than research experience, the T32 program for MDs has been widely criticized for failing to meet its research objectives. Indeed, in 1988, more than 50% of the MDs in T32 training held their awards for less than 12 months, too short a period to have much value as training for research, however valuable it may have been for acquiring clinical skills. (Comparable data for PhDs in T32 programs have not been published, oddly enough; they would make an interesting comparison to the data for MD trainees.)

Dissatisfied with the T32 program for MDs, the NIH Director's Office recently set up an intramural NIH Task Force on training programs chaired by Claude Lenfant, director of NHLBI; its 1989 report, "Review of the NIH Biomedical Research Training Programs," recommended that T32 awards be made for no less than 2 years, with possible extensions to 3 or 4 years, and that competitive renewals be much more rigorously reviewed with respect to their provision of research training. These recommendations were put into action by the acting director of NIH.

In defense of T32s for MDs, Daughaday (1970) had pointed out how valuable such training can be if the awardees are exposed to scientifically trained mentors, but Kunkel (1962) and Kipnis (1979, 1983), among many others, had questioned how rarely this ideal is actually attained. Although fewer than 20% of T32 MDs eventually succeed in winning any type of NIH research grant after completing their traineeships, it cannot be overlooked that, in this large pool of prospective researchers, the most promising individuals have the chance to demonstrate their qualifications for receipt of later, more prestigious, research-productive fellowships.

Fellowship programs (F32) stand in marked contrast to T32 training programs. F32 fellowships are applied for not by medical schools but by individual applicants. Fellows are expected to work under the guidance of research-minded supervisors. F32s are 2-year awards that can be extended to 3 years.

It is important to stress some of the key differences between the T32 and F32 programs, both of which are competitive on a national level. The T awards are reviewed by the IRGs of the several ICDs, which have disease-oriented missions;

the F awards, by contrast, are reviewed by the IRGs and the DRG, which are project-oriented. Accordingly, the criteria for gaining approval by these two different sets of IRGs differ in that the ICD review groups can be said to be more interested in the development of investigators out of a large pool of potential researchers, while the DRG review groups focus more sharply on the content of the research proposal. F32 Fellowships are considered to be more prestigious than T32 traineeships, because they are competed for and evaluated on a national rather than a local level. Nevertheless, it is interesting that the number of T32 applications by MDs has remained rather constant, at an average of 226 per year since 1977, while F32 applications by MDs have nearly doubled, from 254 to 489. Table 11–1 presents these data for MDs, along with changes in rates of

Table 11–1 Training (T32) and Fellowship (F32) Applications and Awards to MDs (Including MD-PhDs)

	No. of Applications			Rates		
	Recommended	Approval	Awarded	Approval	Award	Success
Training Awards						
1977	306	250	145	82	58	48
1978	277	235	173	85	74	60
1979	175	133	77	76	58	44
1980	271	248	200	92	81	74
1981	179	162	103	91	63	56
1982	197	190	131	96	69	63
1983	192	184	152	96	83	78
1984	161	146	91	91	62	57
1985	288	276	200	96	72	69
1986	211	191	96	91	50	45
1987	222	219	144	99	66	63
1988	272	257	139	95	54	51
1989	183	178	99	97	56	54
Mean	226		135	94	65	59
Fellowships						
1977	252	214	132	85	62	52
1978	334	279	168	84	60	50
1979	311	264	164	85	62	53
1980	310	269	137	87	51	44
1981	324	267	122	82	46	38
1982	290	253	137	87	54	47
1983	297	270	147	91	54	50
1984	362	326	151	90	46	42
1985	428	384	198	90	52	46
1986	436	401	147	92	37	34
1987	364	345	163	95	47	44
1988	396	376	166	95	44	42
1989	489	472	144	97	30	29
Mean	353		152	90	51	45

Source: Personal communication, Carol Bleakley, DRG, NIH (July 1990).

approval, award, and success; Table 11–2 shows the same data for PhD's. Several conclusions seem clear from these tables:

1. The number of T32 applications for MDs and PhDs is almost identical: 226 ± 50 for MDs and 229 ± 63 for PhDs.
2. Since 1980, after which more than 90% of the T32 applications were approved by the review groups of the ICDs, the award rates were slightly higher for MDs.
3. There have been no apparent time trends in T32 awards since 1980. However, in regard to the F32 program there have been interesting differences and time trends.

Table 11–2   Training (T32) and Fellowship (F32) Applications and Awards to PhDs

	No. of Applications			Rates		
	Recommended	Approved	Awarded	Approval	Award	Success
Training Awards						
1977	352	246	130	70	53	37
1978	289	232	150	80	65	49
1979	255	186	96	73	52	37
1980	298	273	176	92	65	57
1981	135	122	62	90	51	43
1982	181	168	94	93	56	51
1983	210	192	131	91	68	60
1984	171	158	87	92	55	50
1985	261	253	164	97	65	62
1986	160	149	61	93	41	38
1987	180	176	114	98	65	60
1988	235	225	133	96	59	56
1989	244	242	112	99	46	45
Mean	229		116	94	57	50
Fellowships						
1977	1,332	1,165	747	87	64	56
1978	1,463	1,290	876	88	68	60
1979	1,667	1,502	945	90	63	56
1980	1,421	1,277	649	90	51	45
1981	1,474	1,292	485	88	38	33
1982	1,500	1,339	619	89	46	41
1983	1,439	1,296	628	90	49	44
1984	1,452	1,324	543	91	41	37
1985	1,602	1,512	709	94	47	44
1986	1,575	1,478	415	94	28	26
1987	1,468	1,444	700	98	49	47
1988	1,430	1,384	600	97	43	42
1989	1,648	1,588	468	96	30	28
Mean	1,498		645	92	49	44

Source: Personal communication, Carol Bleakley, DRG, NIH (July 1990).

4. The number of F32 applications by PhDs greatly exceeded those by MDs every year since 1977, and while those numbers rose less than 20% for PhDs, they nearly doubled for MDs over these 13 years.

5. Approval rates of F32 applications by the study sections of the DRG exceeded 90% for PhDs after 1978 and for MDs after 1982; but the award rates for the two degree-holder groups were very similar from 1980 to 1988: 48 ± 6 for MDs and 44 ± 8 for PhDs (omitting the data for 1989, when there was a precipitous drop in the award rates of both groups due to the current fiscal crisis). Not to be overlooked is the general decline in award rates from the earlier to the later years for both groups, consistent with the overall decrease in awards for all NIH awards in the last few years.

6. For the F32s, the ratio of applications to awards was 2.32 for both MDs and PhDs. Once again, this is evidence that the scientific merits of the applications of the two groups of degree holders have been judged to be almost identical.

Fellows (MDs as well as PhDs) have been more successful than trainees in winning NIH grants (of any sort) after the termination of these years in training. Table 11–3 shows the number of newly appointed F32 and T32 awardees from 1976 to 1986 and their ability to win NIH grants on termination of their training years. While PhD trainees fared better than MD trainees, all fellows fared better than all trainees. For MD and PhD Fellows the approval and award rates were almost identical.

The time trends shown in Table 11-3 are not encouraging. The total number of newly appointed MD trainees has more than doubled since 1976, but since 1982 it has leveled off at total numbers almost the same as those for PhD trainees. The number of newly appointed MD Fellows has remained stable since 1977, and while PhD Fellows have declined in number somewhat, they still exceed MD Fellows by 4 to 1. The 1989 *NIH Databook* (Table 39) shows that over the 8-year period (1980–1987), the total number (competing and non-competing) of T32 MDs rose from 1,755 to 2,032 and that of F32 MDs rose from 275 to 325. In contrast, T32 PhDs declined in total number from 2,118 to 1,718, and that of F32 PhDs decreased from 1,429 to 1,273 (still a 4 to 1 margin of superiority over F32 MDs).

Start-up Research Awards

With some sense of the difficulties that promising young research-minded MDs experience in obtaining start-up support funds, NIH has recently initiated two programs, the Physician Scientist award (K11) and the FIRST award (R29), neither of which requires previous research experience. The chances of achieving these awards depend heavily on the recommendations of senior members of the

Table 11–3 Eventual Grantsmanship of NRSA[a] Post-Doctoral Fellows and Trainees (1976–86)[b]

| | Fellow (F32 Awards)[c] | | | | | | Trainees (T32 Awards)[d] | | | | | |
| | MDs | | | PhDs | | | MDs | | | PhDs | | |
FY	No.[e]	App.[f]	Award.[g]	No.[e]	App.[f]	Award.[g]	No.[e]	App.[f]	Award.[g]	No.[e]	App.[f]	Award.[g]
76	167	98	65	929	567	418	282	120	64	545	286	189
77	139	90	67	779	461	336	451	189	123	742	371	241
78	138	87	57	669	376	266	658	236	144	909	462	288
79	129	66	44	773	442	309	793	276	164	1,086	501	293
80	153	86	47	764	389	250	884	284	171	1,116	477	266
81	131	74	53	669	328	218	865	255	143	1,044	386	213
82	120	58	35	505	217	132	909	205	121	1,047	357	199
83[b]	135			614			974			988		
84	187			709			992			974		
85	155			540			1,027			948		
86	134			557			988			907		
Summation 1976–82												
Totals	977	559	368	5,088	2,780	1,929	4,842	1,565	930	6,489	2,840	1,689
Approval Rate[f]		57.2			54.6			32.3			43.8	
Award Rate[g]			37.7			37.9			19.2			26.0

[a]Awards made under terms of the National Research Scientist Act (1975), ranging from $17,000 to $30,000 per year, with payback provisions.

[b]Analysis of applications and awards are cut off after 1982, because these later-appointed fellows and trainees may not have had time to finish training before submitting grant applications.

[c]Fellowships are individually applied for and awarded through the DRG peer review process; 2-year appointments are usual and can be extended.

[d]Traineeships are applied for by medical school authorities, and these institutional applications are ICD peer-reviewed; trainees are selected at the local level, not by NIH. Over these 10 years, 55% of MD trainees terminated training in 1 year or less.

[e]No. = numbers of fellows/trainees newly appointed in the designated fiscal year.

[f]App. = no. of research grant applications (all types of grants) submitted by fellows and trainees (appointed in the designated fiscal years) and approved by IRG's of the DRG or the various Institutes. Approval rate = number approved as a percentage of the number of applications.

[g]Award. = number of research grant applications awarded and funded. Award rate = number awarded as a percentage of the number approved.

Source: Personal communication, Dr. Ronald Geller, Office of the Director, NIH (March 1989).

applicants' medical schools and on the track records of the mentors under whom the awardees will gain this first laboratory experience.

The K11 awards are reviewed by the review groups of the mission-oriented Institutes, whereas the R29 FIRST awards pass under the review of the DRG study sections; this may explain the twofold difference in awards rates shown in Table 11–4. About four times as many R29 awards were made to PhDs as to MDs, with the same award rates (about 25%) to both groups. The K11 award was set up primarily for MDs and has increased steadily in its appeal for young MDs since the program was initiated in 1984. As noted in Chapter 7, the research intentions of the R29 and K11 awardees are heavily weighted toward non-clinical research programs, with only 7.4% and 6%, respectively, designated as programs in Basic POR.

Early Career Awards

The modified Research Career Development award (RCDA or K04), once the most prestigious early career award for young investigators, requires at least 3 years' previous laboratory experience; applications are reviewed by DRG study sections. As seen in Table 11–4, about four times as many awards have been made to PhDs as to MDs, although the two groups achieved about the same award rates. The Clinical Investigator award (K08), designed primarily for MD applicants, requires 5 years' prior research experience; applications are reviewed by the review groups of the funding ICDs. Again, the award rates for MDs and PhDs have been quite similar (Table 11–4).

Table 11–5 shows the time trends on these start-up and early career awards. The K11 awards have remained steady at about 50 new awards per year; the R29 award program has grown rapidly in number since its initiation in 1986, yielding 150 or more experienced researchers per year as each award terminates; the K08 program has stabilized at about 100 exiting scientists per year; the RCDA program (K04) seems to be phasing out, both for MDs and for PhDs.

MD-PhD Programs

Double-degree programs have been in existence for many years, but only on a small scale until NIH launched its Medical Scientist Training Program (MSTP) in 1963 at three U.S. medical schools (Duke, New York University, and Einstein). At present, the MSTP exists in 29 medical schools, and about 700 candidates are currently making their way along this 6- to 7-year track toward the receipt of MD and PhD degrees.

The MSTP is run by the National Institute of General Medical Sciences (NIGMS), which pays all enrollees their tuition costs, living-cost stipends, and some laboratory expenses for 6 years. The selection of candidates is left entirely in the hands of admission committees at each school; each local program is reviewed every 5 years by a site-visiting group of outside (non-NIH) scientists.

In general, the candidates spend the first 2 years with medical school class-

Table 11—4 Start-up and Early Career Development Awards: Applications and Award Rates for MDs and PhDs in FY 1987–89

Activity	MDs			MD-PhDs			PhDs		
	No. of		Award Rate	No. of		Award Rate	No. of		Award Rate
	Applic.	Awards		Applic.	Awards		Applic.	Awards	
K04[a] Modified RCDA	102	38	37%	27	13	48%	422	172	41%
K08[b] Clinical Investigator Award	656	264	40	89	44	49	40	17	43
K11[b] Physician Scientist Award	332	170	51	8	4	50	14	9	64
R29[a] FIRST Award	1,208	301	25	264	83	31	5,087	1,150	23

[a]Applications reviewed by DRG Study Sections prior to decisions on funding by appropriate Institute Councils.
[b]Applications reviewed by ICD Study Sections prior to decisions on funding by their Councils.
Source: Personal communication, Brenda Grimes, Division of Research Grants, Reports Analysis and Presentation Section (June 25, 1990).

Table 11–5 New NIH Awards for Development of Independence in Biomedical Research (K and R29 Awards) (1977–89)

		1977	1978	1979	1980	1981	1982	1983	1984	1985	1986	1987	1988	1989	Estimated Annual Output[c]
K04[a] Research Career Development Award	MD[b]	52	45	47	33	22	32	16	32	26	13	21	13	17	20
	PhD	110	158	126	130	82	111	86	92	89	45	63	68	41	
	Other	7	4	2	3	1		4	3	2	3	3	3	2	
K08[a] Clinical Investigator Award	MD[b]	16	36	29	62	47	42	49	86	111	87	118	97	94	100
	PhD	1	1		1		4	3	2	9	8	5	9	3	
	Other	1	3	2	2	1		3	4	4	6	1	2	1	
K11[a] Physician Scientist Award (Individual)	MD[b]								33	52	38	66	58	50	50
	PhD								1	1	0	2	4	3	
	Other								3	5	6	8	4	10	
R29[b] FIRST Award	MD[b]										33	87	140	157	150
	PhD										20	352	465	333	
	Other										4	10	20	12	

TOTALS: All degrees: annual average, FY77–84 = 218   All degrees: annual average, FY86–89 = 651
MDs[b] only: annual average, FY77–84 = 75; MDs 34% of total   MDs[b] only: annual average FY86–89 = 275; MDs[b] = 42% of total

[a]Annual number of new awards (type 01) for 5 years' support. Previous postdoctoral research experience required: K04 (5 years), K08 (3 years), K11 and R29 (none).

[b]Includes MD-PhDs.

[c]Estimated annual outputs: for K04, K08, and K11 = total no. of MDs[b] (FY84 through FY89) divided by 6
for R29 = total no. of MDs[b] in 1988 and 1989 divided by 2.

Sources: DRG, NIH (Robert F. Moore, April 1989, and Brenda Grimes, June 1990).

mates in the curriculum of that school; then a minimum of 3 years on a research project under the supervision of (usually) a pre-clinical scientist-mentor, culminating in a thesis; and finally, 1 year in the medical school clinical curriculum, on completion of which both degrees are awarded. For most candidates, it has been necessary to lengthen the PhD part of the program to 4 years, which means that non-NIH funds must be found to pay the tuition charges and living costs of the seventh year.

The administrations of the 29 MSTP-sited schools are pleased with this program, and why not? Positions in the program are avidly sought by some of the best students among those aiming at a medical education, and especially by those who profess a dedicated interest in a research career. Naturally, the economics of the program is a compelling feature—6 or 7 cost-free years under well-known scientists in research-rich environments, compared to the escalating costs of 4 years of medical education for those pursuing the MD degree alone. The total cost per MD-PhD graduate is said to approximate $200,000, and more than 2,000 individuals have passed successfully through the MSTP.

It is dismaying to find that the outcome of the MSTP has not been charted by NIH or by any of the schools in which the MSTP has been sited. Thus, there are no hard data nationally on how many candidates dropped out in mid-course or opted to take only one degree rather than both; or on how many graduates chose to complete their medical educations by enrolling as house officers and residents; or how many went into practice or left research for an entirely different career (administration, public affairs, government, industry, etc.); or how many settled down for a life's work in medical schools or research institutes, and in what departments; and, most important of all, how much and what kind of scientific productivity each graduate demonstrated as an independent physician-scientist.

Lacking such data, locally as well as nationally, the administrators at the 29 schools and at NIGMS are flying blind on the entirely understandable presumption that these very talented young people cannot be doing badly—in fact, are probably outperforming their competitors for tenured posts, promotions, and other prizes. Granted the likelihood that this presumption is valid, it would still be useful to know not just that the program has produced many copies of a good product, but what kind of product it is and what purposes that product serves. Anecdotal information abounds, and it is all believable. No matter what career paths are eventually pursued, these individuals are better prepared to follow those paths by having earned both degrees. Furthermore, the environments in which they settle down are undoubtedly well served by the presence of individuals with this broad training.

Even more uncertain is the worthiness of the many other non-NIH funded MD-PhD programs that are said to exist at these same medical schools and at others. In terms of numbers of candidates, there is some evidence from my GCRC Survey (see Chapter 10) that at least an equal number of non-MSTP candidates are undergoing double-degree training—i.e., another 700 individuals. But there are no reliable statistics on these individuals, either in the AAMC

Faculty Roster or in the AMA Physician Masterfile. It is worrying that hard data on the effectiveness of these non-NIH programs also are lacking.

To demonstrate that this kind of product evaluation can be carried out, however laboriously, I made a MEDLINE search in 1990 of the research publications of 82 graduates of MSTP programs in three research-intensive medical schools. These individuals had attained staff appointments as assistant, associate, or full professors (or equivalent status in non-academic sites). Their names and curricula vitae were provided by the three schools' program administrators; these data were used to identify each individual correctly by matching worksites and research training with the publications found in MEDLINE. A total of 754 authors' abstracts were carefully analyzed as described in Chapters 5 and 8 for the 3-D Survey, the CC Survey, and R01 Survey. Table 11–6 presents the results. The main conclusions are that 75% of the publications of these 82 MD-PhDs were focussed on non-clinical research and that only 9% of the publications involved either Basic or Applied POR. Of the 82 double-degree graduates, only 11 were engaged mainly in some type of clinical research and only 2 in Basic POR.

Table 11–6 Analysis of Research Publications of 82 MD-PhDs after Reaching Career-Positions

	Institution A	Institution B	Institution C	Totals
No. of graduates in career positions	26	28	28	82
Graduation years	1978–84	1975–82	1980–87	
Less than 2 years' house staff experience	5	2	9	16
RESEARCH DIRECTIONS OF INDIVIDUAL GRADUATES				
Non-Clinical				
Mainly	13	17	14	44
Exclusively	8	10	7	25
Clinical (any of seven categories)				
Mainly	3	4	4	11
No. who published				
More than one article in basic POR	1	0	1	2
More than one article in applied POR	0	3	1	4
NUMBER OF PUBLICATIONS OF ALL GRADUATES COMBINED				
Total	192 (100%)	356 (100%)	206 (100%)	754 (100%)
Non-Clinical	147 (77%)	259 (73%)	159 (77%)	565 (75%)
Clinical	45 (23%)	97 (27%)	47 (23%)	189 (25%)
Basic POR	6 } (5%)	22 } (14%)	5 } (5%)	33 } (9%)
Applied POR	4 }	28 }	6 }	38 }

Since this analysis was not carried out randomly across all 29 schools in the MSTP, the results cannot be generalized to the entire program. But they do prove that such an inquiry can be launched and successfully completed, given sufficient data to allow correct identification of authors in the MEDLINE database. Whether the authorities, either locally or at the NIH, think that the results of such a survey of the entire MSTP would be interesting and useful is hard to guess; but I believe that the relevant congressional committees would value knowing what this expensive program has produced. Clearly, someone must decide, sooner or later, whether the best and the brightest should have a free ride as a strong phalanx of non-clinical researchers into the faculties of our medical institutions, with no counterbalancing selection of candidates who lean toward some sort of clinical research.

Training Specifically for POR

There is one, and only one, small program dedicated to training young investigators for a career in POR—namely, the Clinical Associates Program (CAP) funded by the GCRC Branch of DRR. CAP awards are available to young investigators who are motivated toward a clinical research career but who are not yet qualified to apply for K04, K08, or R01 awards. They are similar to F32 fellowship awards in that applicants are proposed by medical school mentors but the awards are competed for nationally; awarding decisions are made by the GCRC Advisory Committee and not by DRG study sections. As noted in Chapter 10, some 30–40 new CAP awards are made each year, but the research directions of the 197 individuals who have graduated from the CAP program have never been evaluated.

Time Trends in the Funding of Research Training

The percentage of money devoted to research training by the NIH decreased from 4.6% of total NIH obligations in 1979 to 3.7% in 1988, whereas funding for research grants increased from 62.4% to 72.3%. Table 11–7 (top) shows that, while the annual growth rate for total obligations has been 8.5% per year and 10.3% for research grants, funds for training have grown much more slowly, at only 5.8% per year.

In view of the emphasis given in the pages above to the mechanisms for support of training by the individual Institutes, it is interesting to note in Table 11–7 (bottom) how much each Institute allocated for training in 1988. Among the (then) 12 Institutes, the percentage of total obligations varied from 2.1% to 4.3% (excluding NIGMS, which is mainly committed to funding non-clinical research grants and to training grants and has no intramural research program). For NIH as a whole, institutional training grants (such as the T32 program) consume more than five times as much money as individual training grants (data not shown, but see *NIH Databook,* 1989 Table 39). This ratio certainly deserves

Table 11–7 Funding of Research Training by NIH (in Thousands of Current Dollars): Changes Over Time (1979–88) and Differences Among 12 Institutes

	Entire NIH				
	1979	% of Total	1988	% of Total	Annual Growth Rate (9 Years)
Total oblig. to 1/RD	3,093,986		6,461,985		8.53%
Research training	143,661	4.6	238,954	3.7	5.82
R&D grants	1,930,511	62.4	4,669,870	72.3	10.31
Intramural research	345,432	11.2	715,039	11.1	8.42

	12 Institutes (FY88 only)						
		Research Projects		Research Training		Intramural Research	
	Total Oblig.	Dollars	%	Dollars	%	Dollars	%
NIA	194,548	117,203	60.2	7,966	4.1	23,526	12.1
NIAID	638,521	421,608	66.0	13,093	2.1	77,604	12.2
NIAMS	147,543	96,529	65.4	6,345	4.3	8,756	5,.9
NCI	1,248,981	665,403	53.3	31,861	2.6	268,251	21.5
NICHD	396,584	241,662	60.9	14,127	3.6	46,244	11.7
NIDR	126,216	60,665	48.1	5,236	4.2	24,161	19.1
NIADDK	534,359	372,383	69.7	21,084	4.0	58,556	11.0
NIEHS	215,439	62,221	29.9	9,003	4.2	59,521	27.6
NEI	224,835	166,946	74.3	5,620	2.5	19,723	8.8
NIGMS	632,624	529,041	83.6	66,372	10.5	788	0.001
NHLBI	965,283	603,861	62.6	39,506	4.1	67,963	7.0
NINCDS	534,483	379,606	71.0	13,929	2.6	59,946	11.2

Source: *NIH Data Book* (1989), Tables 8 and 9.

to be re-evaluated, if indeed the value of institutional training grants is deemed to be out of balance with that of support to individual applicants.

The demand for and supply of new physician-researchers may not be so out of balance as many observers have claimed. Table 11–8 presents a greatly simplified analysis in which many of the numbers can be questioned, although they are the best we have for the current period. Predicting tomorrow's need for physician-scientists has foundered on the question of whether the number of MD researchers we now have is what we really need. While some consider our present research workforce to be too small, others argue for more innovative research by better-funded but smaller numbers of investigators. Table 11–8 presents a zero-growth picture that can be modified upward or downward as changes in demand data (number of job offerings, R&D spending, need for teachers) and supply data (number of scientists produced annually) develop. The lack of concordance between demand and supply, shown in Table 11–8 (bottom right), fails to take into account the number of individuals exiting the MD-PhD programs

Table 11–8 Balance Between Supply and Demand for MDs (and MD-PhDs) in Clinical Research in the United States: Facts and Fantasies

Demand Side (AMA Physician Masterfile Projection)		Supply Side (Annual Inputs)	
a. Total no. of active MDs in the United States	525,000[1]	i. Total no. of U.S. medical school graduates per year	17,000[5]
b. Total no. of MDs claiming research as primary activity	17,000[1]	j. Percentage of active MDs claiming research as primary activity (b/a × 100)	3.2%[1]
c. Attrition rate of active MDs per year	5%[2]		
Therefore, no. of M.D.s needed annually to replenish research ranks (c × b)	850	k. Based on research interests of medical graduates (i × j)	680
Demand Side (NIH-PI Projection)		l. From NRSA programs No. of trainees who get NIH grants	125[6]
d. No. of NIH PIs in Dept. of Medicine Survey (1983)	1,753[3]	No. of Fellows who get NIH grants	50[6]
e. No. of MDs in Dept. of Medicine Survey supported by NIH or other funds (but not as NIH PIs)	3,104[3]	No. of exiting MSTP graduates	125[7]
f. Factor for calculation of total no. of MDs supported for research in some manner (e/d + 1)	2.8[3]	No. of clinical investigator and RCDA awardees (K08 and K04)	100[8]
		No. of exiting physician scientist award programs K11	50[8]
g. Total no. of MDs who were NIH PIs nationally (1987)	4,458[4]	K12	10
h. Total no. of MDs supported for research in some manner nationally (f × g)	12,482	m. From FIRST awards (R29)	125[8]
		Total	585
Therefore, no. of MDs needed annually to replenish research ranks (c × h)	624	*Concordance between demand and supply* Demand varies from 624 to 850 Supply varies from 585 to 680	

[1]Physician Characteristics and Distribution in the United States (1988); and AMA Physician Masterfile for 1988, special tabulations, Dept. of Physician Data Services and prior editions, American Medical Association, Tables A-1 and B-15.

[2]From Table 2.5, 1985 IOM Report 85-06; and from Fig. 3-2, IOM Report 88-08, "A Healthy NIH Intramural Program."

[3]Gentile et al. (1987), p. 24.

[4]Summary of FY1987 NIH/ADAMHA Research Support to U.S. Medical Schools, Charles R. Sherman Office of the Director, NIH (May 1, 1989).

[5]Jonas et al. (1989), Table 5.

[6]NRSA outcome data furnished by Dr. Ron Geller, Office of the Director, NIH (March 1989).

[7]From Dr. Lee Van Lenten, MSTP program director, NIGMS, 1989.

[8]From Lucille Nierzwicki, DRG, NIH (1990).

who are *not* NIH financed (non-MSTP), as well as the number of MDs whose training and early career support are derived from sources other than NIH. If, indeed, there is a justifiable need for more physician-scientists, and if a reasonable number of them can be assured some degree of security for, say, a 10- to 15-year research career, ways must be found to recruit more young medical graduates into research careers. This is the subject of the next chapter.

SUMMARY AND CONCLUSIONS

Young research-minded MDs and PhDs who require further training to become independent investigators are faced with a choice of many training and early career support programs. They must be utterly realistic in evaluating their research goals and personal qualifications, and in assessing the degree of institutional support they will receive in terms of the availability of mentors, space, and protected time.

MDs and PhDs have been almost equally successful in winning T32 training posts and F37 fellowships, as well as FIRST (R29) awards. The fact that far more PhDs obtain these three types of awards is due to the much larger pool of PhDs than of MDs, and not to differences in the scientific worthiness of their applications. Trends over time show a dismaying decline in the number of T32 and F32 awards, and only a small increase in FIRST awards, which reflects the declining proportion of total NIH funding of training awards over the period 1977–88 from 4.6 to 3.7% of the total annual NIH appropriation. Institutional training grants like the T32 program consume five times as much money as individual training grants like the F32 program, a ratio that deserves to be re-evaluated.

The MSTP, which currently supports some 700 candidates making their way through a 6- to 7-year course to a double degree (MD *and* PhD), is assuredly successful in attracting talented young people to a cost-free progression through medical school in research-intensive environments and under the mentorship of senior researchers, mostly in pre-clinical departments, but its effectiveness has not been adequately measured. Toward that end, I performed a non-randomized survey of the publications of all 82 MD-PhD graduates from three prominent research institutions (written after they had become independent of their mentors). It showed that 71 were engaged mainly in non-clinical research and only 2 in Basic POR. Whether this is the most desirable outcome of this very expensive federally funded program should be debated in light of the nation's needs for physician-scientists who are skilled in integrative clinical research.

The funding of training and early career support by the private sector (mainly foundations and industry) may amount to only 10% of that of the NIH, but it is considered helpful out of proportion to its size. A complete, updated listing of such offerings is not available from any central source, but it would be welcomed by all who are involved in counseling aspiring young research-minded candidates.

The need for biomedical scientists in the future has not been successfully measured, and it is by no means certain whether our current research pool is too small or too large. Evidence is presented that, in terms only of number, the size of today's pool is being maintained by the combined outputs of the many training programs now existent. Assessments of personnel needs in terms of quality is another story, with strong views on both sides of the question.

12

Basic POR: Endangered But Essential

The history of POR is that of a series of extraordinary achievements in such fields as infectious disease, metabolism, endocrinology, cardiology, surgery, and immunology (to name only a few)—successful explorations that have led to deeper insights into the nature of human disease and, thus, to major progress in diagnosis, treatment, and disease prevention. Practitioners of POR have been among the leaders in medical education, as well as standard bearers for high-quality research and medical care.

Is that situation now "just history"? In view of the procession of stunning intellectual accomplishments in molecular biology that followed the discovery of the Double Helix, some propose, in all seriousness, that the remaining mysteries in human disease can be solved in the laboratory on fragments of patients more effectively than at the bedside with the cooperation of the whole patient. Have the successes of molecular biology made whole-animal studies so dated that they are no longer useful or even appropriate? When a new technology is invented that overpowers older techniques in its capacity to describe events with great precision at an ever more minute level, rather than by less elegant and less controllable experiments at the whole-body level, do we abandon the older approaches in the belief that the new ones will provide answers to all present and future medical problems?

Or are there problems in medical research that can be successfully addressed *only (or mainly)* through the direct study of whole human beings?

With this nation enveloped in an atmosphere of fiscal uncertainty, we need to set priorities and to establish by open debate the relative values of our various missions—economic, social, and military, as well as research priorities. Since the United States can no longer afford to carry out all the various kinds of research for which we have the capability and skills—from outer space to subatomic particles—can we make a reasonable start on priority setting in the biomedical area by weighing the value of the several types of researchers and their degree of endangerment?

Previous chapters have shown that clinical research (as a whole) is in greater danger than non-clinical research. A major reason for this is that the time that MDs spend in research is increasingly restricted by other departmental obligations. As a consequence, they are turning more and more to those forms of research that promise speedier research results, more assured grant renewals, and a smoother path to promotions and tenure. The study sections of the DRG are decreasingly made up of MDs, and those now being enlisted are increasingly reductionistic in their research experience and outlook. As a result, training grants, fellowships, and new R01 grants are increasingly awarded to applicants who do not plan to engage in integrative research.

Previous chapters of this book have shown that of all types of clinical research, POR is the most endangered. Because of its inherent difficulties and constraints, this research activity earns fewer NIH grants than all other forms of clinical research; this, in turn, means fewer publications and promotions. POR attracts only a small share of training and starter grants, such as the K08, K11 and R29 awards; few graduates of the MSTP devote their careers to clinical research and fewer still to POR. Mentors skilled in POR are less and less in evidence in U.S. medical institutions, as time for POR is eroded by the demands of service responsibilities and as aging takes its toll.

Given the conclusion that, of all biomedical research activities, POR is the most endangered, can a case be made for its essentiality and thus its perpetuation? Is POR facing extinction, or as Fredrickson put it (Powledge, 1987), is it simply undergoing a "painful metamorphosis"? Would the dollars spent on the special resources and specially trained ancillary staff be better spent on other research activities? What are the consequences of abandoning POR?

In addressing these very timely questions, we should clearly draw distinctions between the two forms of POR, applied and basic—Category 2 (management of disease) and Category 1 (mechanisms of disease). It is inconceivable to me that Applied POR will disappear from the scene, but for Basic POR it is not unthinkable.

THE LIKELY SURVIVAL OF APPLIED POR

As new drugs are developed, and as new diagnostic and therapeutic procedures are invented and then perfected in animal studies, they eventually must be shown to be effective and reasonably safe when used in human beings. The typical procedure is to evaluate the innovation by comparing it to an accepted modality of management in everyday use at the time of the trial. For short-term studies, such comparisons are usually performed in relatively small numbers of human beings, either in an in-patient or an out-patient setting, depending on the complexities involved. But for long-term evaluations that simulate what will happen when the innovation is applied to the general public, and where the question is whether the benefits outweigh the risks of the intervention, very large numbers of subjects are required for observations and tests over periods of months to years.

Thus, Applied POR is the logical last step after preliminary explorations have been completed by pharmaceutical firms and by academics working at the bench and in animal models. The *designing* of clinical trials requires considerable sophistication in biostatistics and in such management matters as monitoring and safety controls, measurements of compliance, and ensurance of the effectiveness of double-blinding procedures. However, the actual *performance* of such trials can often be left in the hands of competent physicians and ancillary staff members, whose main function is to ensure that the rigidly designed protocols are complied with, and that all required forms, questionnaires, laboratory tests, and clinical measurements are completed. Indeed, many trials can justifiably be mounted in settings that need not be research-intensive medical schools, costly GCRCs, or the NIH Clinical Center. However, it should not go unsaid that, when drug trials are supervised by highly skilled research personnel in carefully controlled experimental settings, important observations of unexpected events and phenomena are made that have led to important uses *other than* those for which the interventions were originally designed; and responses have been noted in the human being (both advantageous and deleterious) that could not have been predicted from earlier animal experiments.

Applied POR is likely to endure, however sophisticated the trial managers may be, because it represents to the public and to Congress the payoff that justifies the expenditure of tax monies for the development of new drugs and devices. Applied POR meets all criteria for justifying its continued support; its end results are eminently desirable for assurance of continued medical progress. Indeed, the costs to society of *not* performing these final tests would be unbearable. The conclusion that Applied POR is thriving (even in these days of fiscal squeeze) is supported by comparing FY1989 NIH expenditures for clinical trials ($500 million) with new R01 grants for Basic POR ($35 million) and by the growing recognition in the pharmaceutical industry that it must assume a larger share of the costs of clinical drug trials (Vagelos, NAS-IOM Forum, 1990).

THE ESSENTIALITY OF BASIC POR

For those who have had extensive experience in Basic POR, and who look on it as basic research whenever it is exploratory work undertaken in an atmosphere of uncertainty, this research activity is considered to be essential to the continued progress of medical knowledge and understanding. That essentiality will be defended on four fronts.

1. There is not now, nor theoretically will there ever be, a perfect animal model for any of the major human diseases, most of which are multifactorial in nature. This does not overlook the fact that much has been learned and will continue to be learned by experiments conducted in normal laboratory animals, such as drug kinetics, toxicities, and modes of action.

But how "normal" is a laboratory animal? More often than not, such animals are pure-bred for genetic features that make them useful to the experimenter.

They are maintained under rigidly controlled conditions that best suit the anthropocentric viewpoints of their keepers. I am reminded of the story of the Rockefeller Swiss mice. For years their respiratory ailments were taken for granted as being normal, but when Dubos and his colleagues abolished those infections in the late 1950s by raising that strain under superclean (but not sterile) conditions, they found themselves working with a metabolically and immunologically different (though genetically identical) mouse strain (Dubos and Schaedler, 1960).

Unlike pure-bred laboratory animals, human beings are anything but genetically homogeneous. In addition, they live under a wide variety of environmental conditions, quite unlike those of an ideal animal care facility, and are challenged daily by a host of different pathogenic organisms and substances. By far the largest percentage of NIH support for new R01s in clinical research is awarded to applicants for studies of animal (or microbial) models of human disease (Category 4). Yet, most experienced investigators realize that animal models of arteriosclerosis, diabetes, hypertension, and cancer are different in important ways from the human conditions they are intended to simulate. Indeed, one of the significant discoveries arising from the new genetics is recognition of the heterogeneity of genetic abnormalities found in disease conditions that appear clinically to be homogeneous.

2. As Dubos emphasized in 1959, new human diseases will continue to appear and be recognized (AIDS is a compelling recent example); tame old pathogens will turn virulent (and vice versa); industry will continue to confront human beings with new environmental challenges; and population pressures will give rise to different economic, social, and behavioral problems in different parts of the world. Only the study of humans can properly address these challenges to the well-being of future generations of the human race.

3. Our rapidly growing understanding of the human genome will demand that the information gained through description of the gene be translated into real-life, real-time functional terms. The triumphs of the new genetics cannot be realized by gene mappers alone. They must take as partners in research those integrationists who are trained to close the loop between the hard-won understanding of human characteristics and their genetic determinants. (Weatherall's 1982 description of the Mediterranean anemias is an excellent example of such an achievement.) Closing the loop between studies in genes and in human disease will depend on the work of highly sophisticated practitioners of Basic POR.

4. New insights in human physiology and behavior, both normal and abnormal, can come only from those who are trained to recognize unusual phenomena in a whole organism. Recognition of the research opportunities presented by human disease requires broad medical training and wide clinical experience. But while clinical acumen is essential, it is not sufficient. The astute clinician who also is research-minded is prepared to ask "why" and "how," as well as "what," and is capable of designing experiments that address these deeper questions.

Thus, Applied POR will certainly continue to thrive. It represents the final and essential step in certifying that a given innovation in the management of disease is safe and effective. *Basic POR, on the other hand, is in danger of being abandoned unless those in leadership positions in academic medicine come to understand that the mechanisms of human disease must be explored in humans. Animal models can never tell the whole story; predicting human medical problems in the future is highly uncertain, and there are no road maps that can lead the investigator in a well-defined way from the 30 billion base pairs of the human genome to an understanding of the complexities characteristic of human function and behavior.*

THE OBJECTIVES OF POR ARE NOT OUTMODED

It has been tempting to make the case for Basic POR by reciting a few of the signal successes in this particular arena of clinical research, as DeKruif did so compellingly in 1926 in *Microbe Hunters*. But however admirable those advances have been in concept and in performance, to rest the argument on that record misses the point of the question. The POR of earlier times was made possible by physiologic and biochemical methodologies that over the years have become ever more accurate and dependable, but in terms of the power to probe smaller and smaller biologic entities, they have been rendered old-fashioned by the newer technologies of molecular biology. Is the fact that so many major medical problems remain unsolved today due to a lack of human ingenuity, or to the complexity of the problems, or to a dependence on tools for seeking solutions that are too blunt? That important problems remain unsolved might lead us to the conclusion that the tried-and-true methods of physiology, metabolism, nutrition, and endocrinology are not up to the task. Or that they haven't been fully utilized by researchers whose time for research is being increasingly constrained. Or that workers in Basic POR have failed to take full advantage of new technologies—not only those of molecular biology, but also those of physical chemistry, immunochemistry, and radiation biology, to name only a few.

The essentialities of POR—both Basic and Applied—are more obvious today than ever. Even if researchers in these areas have been slow in modernizing their technical approaches, it is nevertheless increasingly clear that the *objectives* of POR are critically important to medical progress.

Therefore, studies in humans must be encouraged. Indeed, they must enjoy far greater support than they have today. More researchers in this field are needed, and they must be prepared to take advantage of all modern laboratory techniques. *Recognizing the essentiality of rigorous experimental training, clinically wise MDs and technically wise PhDs must form partnerships in research—each with their special brand of expertise, with equivalent career opportunities, and with joint responsibility for training successive generations of MDs and PhDs who will work together in all types of clinical research.*

SUMMARY AND CONCLUSIONS

The case has already been made that, of all forms of clinical research, Basic POR is the most endangered. It is expensive, it is difficult and slow, and in the competition for training and early career awards and for R01 support, it has lost ground to other forms of research to an ominous degree.

Applied POR, on the other hand, is assured of strong support. As new drugs, devices, and therapeutic methods continue to be developed, the means for testing their efficacy and safety must remain in place. Much of this kind of clinical research can be adequately performed at non-research-intensive sites, rather than in such highly specialized sites as the NIH Clinical Center or in the 74 GCRCs.

There are at least four reasons why Basic POR must be supported, even more strongly that at present. First, there will never be a perfect animal model for the major diseases facing us today and in the future. Laboratory animals are genetically homogeneous and are environmentally protected, unlike man, who comes out of genetic heterogeneity to live in a hostile environment. Second, nature can be counted on to present man with new diseases eternally, and industry will continue to produce new challenges. The medical problems of tomorrow simply cannot be predicted. Third, our growing understanding of the human genome demands that these reductionist advances be translated into functional terms of whole animal physiology and metabolism by physician-scientists who are skilled in integrative research methods. And fourth, only those scientists who are trained to recognize unusual and unexpected phenomena in a whole organism can appreciate the research opportunities presented to them by human disease and be prepared to design experiments in humans that take advantage of those opportunities.

If the formerly useful methodologies of Basic POR have been rendered old-fashioned by recent developments in molecular biology, the *objectives* of POR, both Basic and Applied, remain as critical to medical progress as ever before. Modernizing the technical approaches of POR can best be achieved by MDs forming working partnerships with patient-oriented PhDs.

13

How to Produce an Integrative Physician-Scientist

I argued in the last chapter that POR must be vigorously pursued, and demonstrated in Chapter 11 that training opportunities and early career support mechanisms for MDs are available. These grants are basically bribes to lure research-minded candidates away from what they would otherwise be forced by economic and employment circumstances to do. They offer protected time, the opportunity to work alongside more senior colleagues, and the chance to find out whether they really want to put up with the vicissitudes of a research life and whether they are sufficiently innovative to meet high standards of research activity.

There is no certain way to gauge the number of investigators needed by society to replenish the ranks of those who depart the system and to predict how many will be needed to address the medical problems of the future. A significantly smaller rate of input into the research pipeline through higher selection standards might elevate the quality of the research performed, but at the risk of screening out unconventional candidates and late bloomers. Thus, the safer course is to offer more training opportunities than the system really needs in the expectation that the most promising and talented individuals will identify themselves fairly quickly through their accomplishments. It behooves us now to consider the next pressing question: how can we persuade innovative medical graduates to take advantage of these opportunities?

RECRUITMENT OF MDs INTO CLINICAL RESEARCH

Self-evident are the following barriers to recruitment:

1. Persuading the most talented college students to consider careers in medicine has become increasingly difficult.
   - Fewer college students are well prepared in mathematics and in the life sciences, and their numbers have been decreasing in recent decades.
   - The costs of medical education impose an ever-heavier burden on the middle- and low-income families of prospective students.
   - The uncertainties of financial support for careers in research are driving

research-minded and research-capable college students and medical students away from research, and even away from academic life.

2. Persuading research-minded medical graduates to pursue *clinical* in contrast to non-clinical research also has grown more difficult, as the balance between these two activities in the last decade has tilted markedly toward reductionism and away from integrative research.

   • T32 training grants have failed to produce the number of researchers that was originally expected.
   • Fewer than 5% of the RO1 grants (the hallmark of progress for young investigators) are awarded to MD applicants who seek a better understanding of human biology and human behavior by capitalizing on the research opportunities made possible by observations on human disease.
   • DRG study sections, the first hurdle in winning RO1 grants, are increasingly populated by persons who have little or no experience in POR.
   • Career development awards like the FIRST program and the Physician Scientist award (K11) for promising young research candidates have attracted very few MD applicants who intend to pursue integrative clinical, as distinct from reductionistic non-clinical research.
   • Very few MD-PhD graduates are engaged in clinical research of any type.
   • The publication records of three major clinical departments (medicine, pediatrics, and neurology) indicate that fewer than 40% of those faculty members are devoted to Basic POR.

3. Dedicated time for research is increasingly eroded by the time demands of service to patients.

   • In departments of medicine (presumably the most research-intensive of all medical school departments), half of the department members spend less than 20% of their working time in research.
   • In only a few medical schools do faculty members who have full salary support from their grants enjoy protected time for research. Even MDs who are PIs on RO1 grants must eke out time for research in competition with demands for teaching, service, and administration (not to mention grant proposal writing).

The lesson to be drawn from these discouraging considerations is that recruitment must start earlier and be more persuasive. Those who are most concerned about the deficiencies of modern education urge that remedies be applied from the very start of the school years. In this age of science, it is unpardonable to allow students to leave grade school and college without a basic understanding of the intentions and methods of science and some appreciation of its history. As Tobias (1990) has said of the many college students who choose careers *outside* science, "The first step is a moral and strategic imperative: no college student should be permitted to say 'no' to [introductory] science [courses] without a struggle." To be more persuasive in bringing a significant measure of science to all students, teachers must learn how to make mathematics, chemistry, and physics more relevant to the day-to-day lives of their students and thus to teach more effectively. (Human physiology should be added to Tobias' list; it is pitiful that adults know so little about the workings of their own bodies.)

A number of authors have urged that medical students be exposed as early as possible to clinical research (Di Bona, 1979; Littlefield, 1986; Ross, 1985; Thier, 1980), all of whom emphasized the critically important role that faculty members must accept in promoting that exposure. At Emory Medical School, Daniel Rudman consistently enlisted first-year medical students in the activities of the GCRC of which he was program director (1968–81), and encouraged their continued participation throughout their 4 school years, but if Bickel and Morgan's (1980) and Littlefield's (1986) overly gentle indictment of faculty noninvolvement in this process depicted the norm, the Rudman program was truly exceptional.

The AAMC annually dissects the career expectations of graduating classes of all U.S. medical schools by means of a graduation questionnaire (66% response rate). The percentage of respondents who reply that they expect to be "exclusively or significantly involved in research" increased from 9% in 1979 to 15.6% in 1989; and the percentage of those with a "primary preference for full-time research or academic activities" rose from 20% to 31% over the same period. However unreliable the preferences of graduates may be at graduation time in predicting their eventual careers, the *trends* in replies to the same question indicate the importance of mounting a persuasive recruitment effort during the medical school years.

It is beyond the scope of this book to examine the quality of the educational years *before* medical school, but we cannot pass over the evidence that a period *during* medical school years of "time-out" to undertake a closely supervised research experience has been shown to be beneficial. When in 1928 George Whipple designed the curriculum of a new medical school in Rochester, New York, he planned that medical students and predoctoral students be trained together; in addition, he set up a year-out program for all students that was fully funded by the school. Although objective measures of the effectiveness of this year-out program have not been reported, Young (1981) noted the enthusiasm for clinical investigation that it aroused.

In 1960 Philip Handler and Eugene Stead initiated a year-out program at Duke University Medical School that gave honors students a full year in preclinical laboratories (mainly in cell biology) at no extra tuition expense and without delaying the completion of their medical studies in the usual 4-year period. This program required building new facilities and hiring additional faculty; it was phased out in 1975 in favor of concentrating on the MD-PhD program (MSTP) begun at Duke in 1964. Its early years were described with great enthusiasm by Handler and Wyngaarden (1961) and by Kredich (1978). Though the Duke year-out program has not been evaluated in quantitative terms, it was hailed both locally and nationally as a highly successful educational experiment.

Anecdotal evidence on the benefits of time-out during the medical school years comes from many sources, but two recent reports from the United Kingdom have analyzed the results of year-out programs in a more controlled fashion.

In 1985, Wakeford et al. addressed questionnaires to 378 MDs in the United Kingdom (professors, clinicians employed by the Medical Research Council, former Wellcome Fellows, and a random sample of self-professed research-minded MDs); the response rate was 72%. "Of respondents committed to a research career, 54% of those who reported that undergraduate research had a positive influence on them had decided on this career by graduation, as opposed to only 20% of those who did no research then. Similarly, 54% of those who [did a year-out research program] had chosen a research career by qualification, but only 17% of those without [this experience] had done so."

In 1987 Evered et al. examined the careers of 940 medically qualified professors and readers in the United Kingdom and concluded that those who had taken a year off to do science (leading to a B.Sc. en route to the MD degree) were awarded more grants and had more publications (and more that were frequently cited) than three control groups of U.K. medical graduates.

More on the basis of faith than on hard evidence, the Howard Hughes Medical Institute (HHMI) in 1985 initiated a year-out program (its Cloister Program) to be spent at the NIH by a small number of carefully selected third-year medical students, with full funding by HHMI. (In a third of the cases, a second year-out has been allowed.) To date, some 162 students from 63 different medical schools have taken part in this research program, but it is clearly too early to evaluate its long-term effectiveness in recruiting well-qualified medical students into research careers.

The Sarnoff Society of Fellows for Research in Cardiovascular Science has, since 1979, funded a year-out program for medical students; 10 fellowships are offered each year, and in the first 10 years, 93 fellows enjoyed the research exposure offered by this program. The Pew Charitable Trusts in 1988 began a similar competitive program for four third-year students to work in research on nutrition at Rockefeller University. The Four Schools Physicians Scientist Program in Internal Medicine, initiated in 1989, is more extensive. It makes it possible for two third-year medical students to be selected at each of the participating schools [Duke, Johns Hopkins, Pennsylvania, and Washington (St. Louis)] to enter a fully funded 6-year program of research and clinical training.

In good faith, and perhaps out of a desperate need to recruit medical students into research careers, some commentators have proposed the deliberate formation of two kinds of medical schools—one training MDs for practice and the other stressing research and staffed with role models who attract research-minded students and encourage their participation in research. While many observers disagree with such a policy, a dichotomy of this sort already exists among the 127 U.S. medical schools. Their research intensities span a wide spectrum, from almost zero to millions of dollars spent annually in research. What seems to be lacking, in regard to effective recruitment of students into research, are close personal contacts between faculty and students. Both groups seem overwhelmed by the demands on their time; and the larger the school, the greater the distance between students and qualified mentors.

PhDs in Clinical Departments

Changing Perceptions. PhDs continue to serve an essential training role in the pre-clinical departments of U.S. medical schools. However, in recent years, their presence as members of clinical departments (where they comprise about 17% of the full-time faculty) has not only enlivened the pursuit of biomedical research of those departments but has had an important impact on training at all levels—medical students, residency staffs, and senior clinicians.

In this mix of MDs and PhDs, who are the "real" doctors? This traditional jibe bespeaks the wariness that has traditionally characterized the relationships between PhDs and MDs. Each group considers itself better qualified to be the real doctors, the one to do real science, the other to do the real work of medicine. Such feelings still exist in the form of subtle marks of discrimination, but they will become muted as each group comes to appreciate the strengths of the other and their mutual interdependence.

Evidence has been presented in previous chapters that MDs are becoming increasingly engaged in non-clinical research and that PhDs have become involved, often as leaders, in certain types of clinical research. One stricture still remains. By law, PhDs cannot be held responsible for the care of patients, nor can they undertake research on patients without the collaboration of one or more MDs; non-invasive behavioral research on volunteers by psychologists may be an exception. Thus, non-clinical research is currently undertaken by both MDs and PhDs. Basic and Applied POR must involve MDs as participants, but all other clinical research (Categories 3–7) is currently carried out by PhDs or MDs (and often both in partnership).

It is generally agreed that, through their postgraduate training and postdoctoral years of research experience, PhDs are well equipped to handle the increasing complexities of modern technologies, while MDs are uniquely trained to recognize the complexities of human health and disease, to appreciate the challenges of disease as experiments of nature, and to see the research opportunities that aberrations in human physiology open up to the inquiring medical mind. The converse also is true. Most MDs are inexperienced in the theory and utilization of modern technologies, and many PhDs are little more aware of the wisdom of the human body than are intelligent laymen.

While first- and second-class distinctions are slowly disappearing, certain privileges and jealousies remain. Because MDs have the almost exclusive right to minister to patients, many of them believe that this time-consuming and highly responsible obligation justifies the higher incomes commanded by MDs. But even among PhDs themselves, there are strong hierarchical prejudices. PhDs employed in pre-clinical departments consider themselves to be first-class scientists, and often regard those who accept appointments in clinical departments as second-raters who have abandoned their "guild." And to the extent that MDs in clinical departments withhold leadership roles from their PhD colleagues, the enthusiasm that ought to exist when MDs and PhDs collaborate is likely to be dampened.

Some of our most highly respected medical researchers have watched with admiration the march of biomedical science driven by the complicated technologies most familiar to PhDs, and they have asked whether MDs ought not to concentrate on what they know best (human biology) and leave the tricky details for PhDs. Castle preached that message with sincerity and vigor in 1960, but 3 years later, Wood warned his colleagues of the dangers of denying the power of reductionistic research. Beeson in 1967 predicted that MDs would inevitably lose out to PhDs in competing for the deeper biological truths, and urged them to turn back to fields in which they are pre-eminently and uniquely qualified. By 1981, however, some MDs recognized the special contributions that PhDs can and do make in medical research, and they urged their medical colleagues to join with them in increasingly effective ways (Fishman and Jolly, 1981; Lipsett, 1981). But of course, others set out simply to out-compete the PhDs at their own game, and many succeeded.

PhDs as Assets. Department chairmen evaluate the assets of their departments in terms of staff members, space, and income generation. They count the number of publications in peer-reviewed journals produced by their full-time faculty and the number of research grants (especially from NIH, but also from any other external source) and the attendant overhead costs that are welcomed by their administrators. They take pride in the number of promotions squeezed out the school's promotion committees, as well as the prizes and other accolades bestowed on their colleagues. They also respond gladly to the department members who willingly share in the teaching and administrative duties of their schools, and note the number of faculty members who require no departmental funding. They protect the square feet of laboratory space captured by their staffs, and carefully reckon the amount of income generated for their departments from fees and insurance payments charged for medical and laboratory services to patients. Indeed, all these factors create the image of the department in the eyes of trustees, prospective donors, other universities, and the community of patients served by that facility; and they do not go unnoticed by prospective faculty recruits and applicants to their medical schools and house staffs.

PhDs contribute, each in their own way, to all of these assets *except* for generating income from medical fees. Less visible but no less important services are rendered by PhDs in clinical departments. They take an active part in designing experiments with their medically trained colleagues, in helping to perform them, in analyzing the data achieved, in preparing the reports of those experiments, and in helping to write the grants needed to carry those experiments to the next step. Their expertise lends more than a veneer of sophistication to these tasks.

As shown in our analysis of the MSTP program in Chapter 11, MD-PhDs more often than not are "PhDs in MD clothing," most of whom are engaged in non-clinical research. However, there is no question that their presence in a clinical department can be catalytic and provocative, and indeed image-enhancing.

Constraints on PhDs. Because the PhD cannot be responsible for the medical care of patients and is rarely a major generator of income to the department, he has been discriminated against in promotions to tenured positions and in salary. So long as PhD salaries and laboratory costs are covered by grants from external sources, their appointments remain secure, and their promotions are based on the quality and quantity of their research. Although many PhDs in clinical departments are funded by the grants of their clinical colleagues, it is noteworthy that 27.5% of the 8,038 PhDs in clinical departments of U.S. medical schools in FY1987 were PIs on NIH/ADAMHA grants (Sherman, 1989) compared to 12.2% of MDs (plus MD-PhDs) in those clinical departments. However, if PhDs lose their own grants and cannot generate funds from other sources, it is unlikely that their department chairmen can find the necessary funds to support them for more than a short time, and, since they cannot shift their energies to the clinic, as MDs can, they must leave. To do what? Possibly to accept a teaching post at another university, college, or school, or a position in a profit-making enterprise, or in government, or even in the NIH administration itself.

Because of these uncertainties, and because too many MDs see the PhD more as an adornment than as an absolute necessity in their clinical work, many PhDs in clinical departments fail to get the respect and esteem of the MDs who outrank them. A partial remedy for this insecurity is the dual appointment: PhDs may hold secondary posts (usually unpaid) in a pre-clinical department, in which case they do their share of pre-clinical teaching. Nevertheless, their pre-clinical chairmen may look upon them as adjuncts rather than regular staff members, and deny them the full measure of support that is offered to full-fledged department members. According to the AAMC Faculty Roster System, only 13% of the PhDs in clinical departments held these secondary appointments in 1981 (Fishman and Jolly, 1981); in 1990, this percentage stood at 14% (Whiting, AAMC, personal communication).

Cooperations and Partnerships. The number of PhDs in many clinical departments has increased as MDs have reduced their personal commitments of time to research, squeezed by increasingly heavy demands for service to patients.

The literature is rich in expressions of welcome to these talented individuals into clinical research, and in the recommendation that there be closer partnerships between pre-clinical and clinical departments in an era characterized by increasing team research. What is urged is cooperation, not competition; mutual respect for each other's strengths and competencies; a sharing of departmental duties and obligations and a voice in departmental decision making; equitable career pathways and job security; and recognition of the dependence of each trained group on the other, even in clinical research. It goes without saying that each group must find the time to keep in touch with the latest developments in its field through periodic re-training.

This drawing together of MDs and PhDs, which seems so essential in the face of the increasing complexity of medical diagnosis and management, as well as in laboratory technologies, is growing more common. Note the 2-year course in modern laboratory techiques for MDs at Pittsburgh that is taught entirely by PhDs who are themselves enticed into clinical collaborations through this experience (Lehotay et al., 1982). Note the popular one-semester course in human pathobiology for PhDs at Tufts, guided along Socratic lines by an MD who is head of the division of gastroenterology (Arias, 1989). Note the guidelines of the Association of Medical School Pediatric Department Chairmen for training physician-scientists in that field, stressing the need for cooperation of pre-clinical and clinical chairmen in selecting the most committed MD candidates to work with the best-qualified mentors (Kelch and Novello, 1989).

These heartening new developments have led me to wonder whether young MDs and PhDs are not ideally equipped to train each other. Each group needs to know what can be learned from the other, for their skills are complementary and interdependent. Indeed, the exploration of key medical issues by the two groups working and training together could be an exciting experience. Can MDs and PhDs do together what neither does quite so well alone?

SPECIAL TRAINING NEEDS OF INTEGRATIVE PHYSICIAN-SCIENTISTS

Physician-scientists who concentrate on POR need a special kind of training. Those who specialize in studies on the management of disease (Applied POR) need personal experience in pharmacology, nutrition, physiology, and biostatistics. In contrast, physician-scientists engaged in mechanistic studies of human disease (Basic POR) are asking why certain phenomena occur in the natural course of disease and how certain manipulations (foods, drugs and other environmental influences, physical activity, sleep) affect the whole organism. Thus, Basic POR spans the entire spectrum of medicine and all its subspecialties. The individual researcher will no doubt approach a particular part of that spectrum from his own vantage point of training in one of the subspecialty disciplines. He must become competent in all the laboratory and experimental aspects of that discipline, and be aware of and eager to capitalize on new technologies as they are developed, in order to bring these powerful tools to bear on the questions and hypotheses under test.

What, then, is the best way to train physician-scientists in Basic POR? Given the presently overloaded medical curriculum, with its dearth of scientific underpinning and absence of laboratory exposure, I question whether the best solution is another 3 to 5 years' training in one of the pre-clinical laboratories, aimed at matching the depth and scope of training that PhDs acquire at a considerably earlier age. Is it reasonable and advisable to demand another long period of immersion in modern technologies (after 7 or 8 years of medical education) to acquire familiarity with the language, thought processes, and technical competencies of PhDs, while clinical skills lie fallow?

MD-PhD programs, as they now exist, are certainly not the way to create a Basic POR physician-scientist. The 29 existent MSTP programs have been organized by PhDs and MD-PhDs who are highly competent reductionists; thus, it is not surprising that the graduates of their programs have tended to replicate their mentors' research directions and laboratory skills, with 75–80% of them pursuing *non*-clinical research. But the MSTP has taught us a valuable lesson: the qualities of the mentors determine the qualities of the graduates.

Ross (1985) and Littlefield (1986) asked, why not establish an MD-PhD program specifically designed to produce a clinical researcher? Should one or more MD-PhD programs be set up in which POR mentors produce copies of themselves? No, not good enough.

I propose that a *post-post*graduate program be set up in at least one medical school as a pilot study of, say, 10 years' duration—organized by a team of senior scientists, some of whom are reductionists (biochemists, physiologists, pharmacologists, molecular biologists) and others who are integrationists with demonstrated skills in human metabolism, physiology, nutrition, and behavior. Their jointly agreed-upon program of learning-by-doing would advertise for applications by recently graduated PhDs and by MDs with a minimum of 2 years of house-staff experience. The essential guidelines: that equal numbers of PhDs and MDs be selected as candidates; that the mentors be articulate and dedicated to the success of the program and that they teach by example; that the applicants and mentors all have an avowed interest in research on whole human beings; and that the candidates *teach each other* by working together as partners on research *themes* (not mini-projects) of their own joint devising under the supervision of their PhD and MD advisers.

Young MDs and PhDs have much to teach each other from two different vantage points. It is my personal experience that PhDs can rapidly learn the essentials of human physiology and behavior, and that MDs can quickly become conversant with experimental design and modern technologies. Flexibility in working arrangements should be encouraged in order to maximize the transmission of knowledge and skills among the candidates.

"Graduation" would occur on completion of research programs deemed by the integrative and reductionist organizers to signify the development of independent researchers who are now qualified to seek and win RO1 (or equivalent) external funding. There would be no tuition fees; stipends and allowances would fall in the same range as those that are compatible with local salary levels of third-year medical residents. Since PhDs would not become physicians, nor would MDs become PhDs, doubling of degrees would not be the goal. Perhaps an M.Sc. in clinical research would serve to document successful passage through this novel experience. The most desirable outcome of this training experience would be independent integrative scientists who have learned the enormous benefits of cooperation with a complementary breed of graduate student, and who thereafter would seek and find partners in research, working in tandem and continuing to learn from each other.

This program represents a unique combination of learning and researching that for each candidate could last as long as 5 years. At the end of that time the graduates would be (on average) 29 and 33 years old (PhDs and MDs, respectively), full-fledged researchers eligible for positions as assistant professors (at the least) in clinical departments. Indeed, they would constitute the best-trained participants in clinical research centers in the most research-intensive institutions.

Funding of such an experimental program should optimally be undertaken by a foundation in the private sector, perhaps in collaboration with industry (pharmaceutical, biotechnology, or food). The full cost of bringing such candidates up to the competence level of independent investigators need not exceed the monies that senior investigators now allocate from their own grants to the presence in their laboratories of young investigators at the start of their research careers—$50,000 to $60,000 per person per year.

SUMMARY AND CONCLUSIONS

Training opportunities for MDs who are research-minded but typically undertrained scientifically do, in fact, exist. How, then, can we persuade some of them to consider undertaking careers in POR, the single activity in clinical research that is most endangered? The barriers to recruitment of young MDs into academic life generally and into POR specifically are numerous and daunting but can be overcome if POR physician-scientists appreciate the necessity to launch recruitment efforts early, even in the college years, and certainly from the first year of medical school education. Inquiring individuals must be identified as early as possible and be made aware of the many advantages and personal gratifications of careers in POR. The success of this campaign will be greatly enhanced by the presence of teams of POR scientists made up of MDs and PhDs who demonstrate their expertness in experimental design and in the application of modern technologies.

Large numbers of PhDs have joined clinical departments and are taking part in clinical research programs, even as PIs on RO1 grants. On the other hand, medically qualified department members are increasingly burdened by clinical responsibilities and the need to generate income for their departments by providing medical service to patients; whether the number of hard-core MD researchers is ebbing or waning is not known. Because of the important roles that PhDs will increasingly play in forward-looking, innovative Basic POR, their careers in these clinical departments must be made far more secure. They must have promotions and salary rewards that are commensurate with their scientific merits, and they must be treated as first-class partners.

There are special training needs for integrative physician-scientists that will not be fulfilled by any of today's training programs unless POR mentors take a more commanding lead in shaping those programs to the needs of POR. Not a single NIH-funded MD-PhD program aims to graduate integrative physician-scientists, despite the success with which the MSTP has launched MD researchers into reductionist careers. MD-PhD programs in integrative research will be effective only insofar as they are organized by teams of MDs and PhDs with skills in both integrative and reductionist disciplines; serious efforts in that direction should be undertaken.

Even more likely to succeed is a novel proposal to enlist newly graduated PhDs with young MDs finishing their clinical fellowships to work together on themes of POR under the guidance of MD and PhD mentors, *training each other* in their particular skills. A pilot study of such a *post*-postgraduate program deserves serious consideration.

I don't agree. Better to use a seasoned M.D. c̄ a young PhD

14

Stronger Support for POR in U.S. Medical Schools

The endangerment of basic POR—the central theme of this book—has deep roots: in dissatisfaction with the provision of medical care in the United States; in the shortcomings of educational systems at all levels, but particularly in U.S. medical schools; in the waning morale of biomedical researchers who are competing fiercely for funding by the NIH; and in the forbidding economic and social dilemmas facing the United States in these last years of the twentieth century.

In the long term, the health of POR depends directly on the health of American medicine, which in turn depends on achieving at least three re-definitions. First, there is a pressing need to re-define the primary mission of U.S. medical schools. Can the delicate but teetering time-honored balance between education, research, and service be preserved, or must this three-legged stool be re-designed? Our academic medical centers have become top-heavy organizations in which education has taken a back seat to service and research. It is not too soon to question whether the educational activities of U.S. medical schools can usefully be separated from the overwhelming responsibilities of service to the public. Would some separation of the relatively small requirements for education and research from the vast needs for medical services in our gargantuan academic health centers produce a better educational experience for the medical students enrolled in these academic centers?

If top-heaviness has become a drawback, can smallness be defended as a twenty-first-century goal for U.S. medical schools? Indeed, what are the *minimum* numbers of teaching faculty, teaching facilities, teaching beds, and clinics that are required for, say, 100 students per entering class? Given a minimum size that guarantees a critical mass of teaching faculty, will smallness per se lead to a more personalized system with closer contacts between students and teachers, more collegiality among the faculty, better teaching, and even better research?

Second and no less important is the need to re-think the ways in which U.S. medical schools are supported financially. Is it rational to bank an educational system on the spinoffs from research grants and on income generated by medical service to the general public, neither of which is wholly and directly concerned with medical education? In fact, if the smaller resources required for medical education were separated from the vastly more expensive facilities demanded by medical service, might not U.S. medical schools expect to win increasing support from those elements of the private sector that have the most to gain from a better system of medical education? Let me be more specific: I refer to the public and private insurance industries (especially the Medicare system) and those enterprises whose profitability depends on the quality of the graduates of our medical schools (the pharmaceutical, food, and biotechnology industries in particular). And, with a return to smaller and more effective medical schools, might the not-for-profit agencies and foundations resume their critically important support of highly qualified students and young investigators through grants and fellowships?

And third, it is essential that doctors and medical scientists make a serious effort to close ranks with the U.S. public and win back its confidence and moral support. Would it not help to accept a more justifiable wage structure and to reassert (through personal example) the ideals of humanitarianism and kindliness that still motivate young people to apply for admission to medical school even today? If academic MDs made it their policy to take part in some of the activities of the AMA, could academics and practitioners, working together, introduce reforms that focus on cost-efficient prevention rather than costly remedial medicine? Is it not time for Congress (representative of the public) and the biomedical establishment (for-profit and not-for-profit) to draw together and become more effectively informative and constructive?

These long-term issues are a minimum agenda for constructive debate, and not pie-in-the-sky dreams. Can we afford to wait for further dehumanization of the medical care delivery system before we address these matters? Is our leadership capable of convincing us that the eleventh hour is already here?

MEDICAL EDUCATION: GENERAL AND PARTICULAR CONCERNS

General Matters for Faculty Debate

Every medical school seeks to reach some sort of equilibrium among the demands of its three missions—education, research, and service. Yet, the balances achieved more often reflect the impact of community forces, as well as responses to changes in federal laws dealing with physician shortages and maldistribution of health care facilities. Only a few schools have been organized with radically new objectives in mind: Case-Western Reserve with its organ-oriented curriculum, in which clinical and pre-clinical teaching are carefully integrated; Hershey (Pennsylvania) Medical Center with its focus on community medicine, the humanities, and medical ethics; Duke with its compression of pre-clinical instruction into a single year in order to make possible an elective year in research; and McMaster with its focus on the social side of clinical medicine and on learning to weigh the effectiveness of alternative therapies.

In terms of size, most schools have grown like Topsy in reaction to such external forces as the availability of federal monies for enlargement of student bodies, buildings to house them, hospitals in which to offer care to their communities, and funds for all things required for biomedical research. Medical centers are now so large that the various faculties fail to know each other or the nature of each other's work.

A useful step toward collegiality would be for faculties to meet together more frequently, not merely to address short-term crises but also to seek common ground on major objectives; to agree on how to reach those goals considered to be central to the pursuit of education, research, and service; and to define the standards of excellence that each school aims for in all its endeavors. (This would be eminently feasible if schools were smaller in size.)

Three distinctive characteristics, inherent in the ambience of a given medical school, establish the level of regard in which it is held in comparison with others; they need periodically to be debated and re-defined.

1. *Mentorship:* What characteristics are most essential in the teachers, researchers, and clinicians who are responsible for inspiring and instructing young followers?
2. *Leadership:* What qualities and characteristics distinguish leaders from followers? Is the quality of leadership born in a given individual, or can it be acquired? How do leaders differ from mentors?
3. *Quality:* What, specifically, do we mean when we speak of the quality of research or the quality of mentorship? Is quality measurable?

We use these terms without knowing whether we agree on their meanings. Therefore, at the least, an open debate will bring out what is *not* agreed upon. The recent public turmoil over fraud in science has forced faculties to come to agreement on standards of openness, honesty, and behavior. This useful exercise has forced faculty members to define terms and to put it on record that as a community they intend to live up to certain standards. Even if complete agreements on the deeper meanings of quality, mentorship, and leadership—and their implications—are not achieved, the act of laying open the different, seemingly irreconcilable viewpoints will be helpful.

Special Faculty Concerns

Reward Systems (Criteria for Advancement). Having sought some degree of consensus on matters of quality, mentorship, and leadership, faculties need next to consider the reward systems that prevail in their institutions. In earlier days, the highest rewards were bestowed on clinicians—those who were most experienced, had the best grasp of the literature, were articulate in explaining their reasonings and conclusions, and who, because of their personalities, enjoyed the admiration of their patients and colleagues. Then, with the passage of time and the advance of scientific medicine, the clinician-teacher-researcher became the person most admired, envied, and emulated. Today it is generally accepted that such "triple threats" no longer exist. While a few faculty members display great talent in two of these three areas, most are satisfied to be judged competent in just one of them. And now a fourth dimension of skill must be added—that of the administrator, a category that includes department chairmen and deans, as well as hospital managers.

By what criteria do faculty members weigh the merits of their clinicians, teachers, researchers, and administrators? How do promotions committees decide whether an expert clinician deserves promotion to the next academic grade, in preference to a superb teacher or a highly competent researcher?

It would seem obvious that a single yardstick is of little help in comparing the merits of individuals in different disciplines and activities. Clearly, clinicians should be compared to other clinicians, and not to researchers; teachers to other teachers; and so on—each with a set of criteria that is most appropriate to that individual's professional activity.

This entirely obvious precept rarely prevails. There are very few institutions in which faculty members working in each of the three medical activities (education, research, and practice) evaluate each other as a unit, each making its own decisions on merit separately from the other two. Today, as an heirloom of the golden era of biomedical research in the 1950s and 1960s, most non-administrative professionals are measured against a criterion that is appropriate for researchers but not for clinicians or teachers: prominence based on research productivity. The degree of prominence is judged in terms of success in winning external grant support through peer-review processes; by numbers of publications and the frequency with which they are cited by other authors; by invitations to serve on peer-review groups and to hold named lectureships in other institutions; and by membership in elitist societies like the National Academy of Sciences, the Association of American Physicians, and the American Society for Clinical Investigation. A yardstick based on research productivity certainly is appropriate for all researchers, but it is a highly misleading and unjust measure of the worthiness of teachers and clinicians. And even among researchers, research productivity should be measured with an understanding that reductionist research proceeds at a very different pace from integrative research, and with different precisions and constraints. In an ideal world, researchers in Basic POR will be judged in comparison with each other, and not with clinical trials experts, epidemiologists, animal modelers, or molecular biologists.

A case can be made that medical schools will be more productive, more harmonious, and more attractive to prospective staff members if rewards (esteem, promotions, salaries) are bestowed on each of the four elements of the faculty in accordance with criteria for advancement that are appropriate to each particular activity. Reforms in today's bizarre value system can be achieved only if consensus is reached through general faculty discussion.

Departmental and Postgraduate Degree Barriers. Historically, there has been a regrettable, though understandable, coolness between MDs and PhDs in U.S. medical schools. This aloofness has resulted from differences in educational backgrounds and values, in career objectives, in disproportionate hiring patterns, and in differing salary levels.

Arguments and evidence have been presented in Chapters 5, 7, 11, and 12 for the merits of close cooperation between pre-clinical and clinical departments—in teaching, in research, and even in providing service to patients. With the growing complexity of medicine, teamwork has become the order of the day, and single-author reports have become a rarity. In fact, multiple authorship is almost the rule. Co-authors with various postgraduate degrees work in different departments, and even in different institutions and countries.

When it becomes more widely recognized that these variously trained professionals have much to offer each other in work skills, teaching opportunities, and research interests, tribal antagonisms will fade away. However, this will not happen unless equitable arrangements are made for rewarding all players on the basis of their competence, skills, and contributions.

Why are salary levels and tenure not based solely on merit? Does the MD's ability to generate service income justify a higher salary level than that paid to PhDs of comparable scientific competence? In considering the promotion of a PhD in a clinical department, should not that individual's value in his partnership with his MD colleagues be the determining factor in setting salaries and awarding promotions? Is it reasonable for MDs to question the promotions and salaries of their PhD partners on the basis that PhDs have no responsibility for life-and-death decisions?

How ideal it would be if the resources of all departments and all participants were pooled and then apportioned to faculty members on the basis of individual merit, without regard to departmental boundaries, postgraduate degrees, and perceived prerogatives. Such utopian efforts in the past have regularly been hindered by the market forces of supply and demand, with talented persons in short supply demanding and getting more favorable treatment. Here is one more argument for smaller and more collegial medical schools in which intolerable imbalances might be minimized through faculty agreements on salaries and ranks based on merit. No such policy is operative in U.S. medical schools today, although it worked well for nearly 10 years at the new medical school in Hershey, Pennsylvania, until it, like so many others, became a big business enterprise.

The opening pages of this chapter were devoted to a few general considerations that merit serious long-term attention, for if attention is not paid to such issues as medical school size and collegiality, faculty consensus on basic issues of quality and leadership, territorial warfare between MDs and PhDs, and the inequities of present-day reward systems, then it may be a waste of time and effort to address the urgent problems now faced by Basic POR (and their possible remedies).

However, I have faith that these general issues will be faced and satisfactorily addressed. The remainder of this chapter is devoted to new strategies and possible solutions at the U.S. medical school level. Chapter 15 will take up issues that must be faced by the NIH.

THOUGHTS FOR THE LEADERSHIP IN U.S. MEDICAL SCHOOLS

The earlier chapters of this book have presented the evidence that Basic POR is declining in quantity and quality (and have discussed the reasons for these changes), but I have argued that this category of clinical research will be increasingly essential in the future as new understandings gained at the molecular level demand translation and application in the whole organism. It is my hope that leaders in U.S. medical schools will become increasingly alarmed over the current downgrading of POR and the threatened disappearance of POR scientists in their schools and will attempt to face the issues discussed in the following section.

Deans for Clinical Research

A major reason for maintaining the GCRC system is that GCRC units make possible the performance of Basic POR of high quality and fastidious performance. Applied POR, on the other hand, can usually be undertaken at non-GCRC sites—that is, in special treatment centers like intensive care units, in subspecialty outpatient units, and even on general wards and general clinics. Applied POR is focused on management-of-disease issues: evaluations of new drugs, new procedures, new diagnostic tests, and new devices. In contrast, GCRCs, which are more appropriate for studies on the mechanisms of disease, offer special facilities for meticulous observations and measurements in patients who are admitted at no cost for studies whose durations are not constrained by the economies imposed on hospitals today by the Medicare system. In addition, they offer a special environment, away from the hustle and bustle of general wards and general outpatient clinics, and are staffed by nurses and dietitians trained to carry out the meticulous observations that Basic POR requires.

Basic POR investigators need strong institutional support to meet the challenges posed by conflicting departmental concerns over staffing, budgets, space requirements, promotions, and recruiting of patients as well as of staff. To meet these demands, the GCRC branch has dictated that the PIs on GCRC grants be the dean (or an equivalent authority), rather than a department chairman, so as to prevent the monopolizing of GCRC facilities by any given medical specialty. This chain of command keeps these units general in scope and encourages their use by all clinical elements of the medical center.

Some deans, burdened by a host of time-consuming responsibilities, duties, and distractions, have recognized that POR workers have a special, critically important need for strong institutional support, and have delegated this particular responsibility to an associate dean for research and, in a few cases, to an associate dean for *clinical* research. That associate dean is conversant with all the clinical research activities of the school and is encouraged to concern himself with long-term plans for the research most appropriately performed by that school's faculty mix; to organize the recruiting of new staff members whose records indicate their continuing interest in performing some type of clinical research; to arbitrate in matters of space allocations for these researchers; and to oversee the deliberations of the promotion committees that so importantly control the destinies of the young investigators recruited into such studies. Deans for research who are well informed about all the research activities of their schools can stand up to the demands of department chairmen and hospital managers, and turn potential conflicts into support for the needs of their clinical research teams.

A dean for clinical research should be preferably an MD who has spent productive years in some form of clinical research and is prepared to assist less experienced colleagues who show talent and interest in any area of clinical research. In view of the jeopardy in which Basic POR finds itself today, this particular category of clinical research will be a major concern for such a dean.

Much more than an expediter of grants and grants management, an associate dean for clinical research should be the key middleman in dealings with the NIH, interested foundations, and prospective donors. The program director of a local GCRC is not, in my view, the most appropriate person to be the dean for clinical research.

Institutional Support for Basic POR Scientists

Many of the persons who currently oversee the activities of GCRCs as program directors also serve as subspecialty division heads (as in endocrinology, hematology, or diabetes). Such leaders have emphasized the importance to their units of being part of the main information stream in their schools; being a division head and meeting frequently with other division heads serves that purpose. But there are other ways to be influential in decisions that affect the health and prosperity of Basic POR. A few GCRCs enjoy departmental status, and their directors meet regularly with departmental chairmen. Some directors sit on the executive committees of their faculty, others on their hospital boards. Some are included on promotions and search committees. Being in the information stream signifies involvement in such major activities as recruiting for new faculty appointments and having a voice in faculty promotions and space allocations. Such added responsibilities are not urged in order to give prestige or power to the program directors. Being in the information stream means that the program director has a voice (and often a vote) in arguing for the choice of a new faculty member with personal experience in Basic POR.

For GCRC units to prosper, it is essential that the job of program director be made more attractive than it is today. The program director must have protected time in which to perform Basic POR himself, free from many of the routine departmental duties that most members of the department must assume. Being a role model and mentor is the director's most important responsibility to his unit; serving those functions requires protected time.

To that end, the director must be free of the requirement to earn part of his income through service to patients; his entire salary must be provided out of GCRC and institutional funds. This objective is thwarted today by the NIH. The GCRC Branch has ruled that it will provide the director with no more than a half-salary and that the other half must come from other sources. The Branch rationalizes this ruling by saying that it allows the director time in which to perform high-tech laboratory studies that will ensure his winning an RO1 grant! If the Branch fails to abandon this ruling, which seriously curtails the director's effectiveness as the leader of his unit, the financial burden of providing the second half of the director's salary must be assumed by the institution. The director must be fully salaried in order to protect his time for the performance of and leadership in Basic POR.

Why is it that protected time is a prerequisite for *all* performers of Basic POR? Basic POR is the most time-intensive of all types of clinical research. Personal contact with research patients cannot be delegated to technicians, field workers, or to the other assistants who play such useful roles in performing less time-intensive forms of clinical research. Major users of GCRC facilities as well as the program director have responsibilities and obligations for work and workers in their own laboratories, and for obtaining the funds to support that work. To the extent that major users' salaries are not provided entirely from their own research grants, such shortfalls must be met by departmental or institutional funds. Time for Basic POR must not be eroded by departmental needs for income generation through service to patients.

The matter of special funding arrangements for POR workers will be a major task for the dean for clinical research, and will require diplomacy and ingenuity in winning a significant share of the discretionary funds dispersed by the dean's office. This case can be won only if the research dean appreciates the unusually heavy time demands required for Basic POR.

In the near future, it may be wise to contemplate cost sharing for Basic POR between NIH and the host institution, especially if congressional appropriations to the GCRC Branch fail to keep up with inflation. One way to accomplish this is to seek endowment funds specifically earmarked for Basic POR, for this is an activity that seems understandable and appealing to prospective private donors. Of all appeals for endowment funds, that for Basic POR seems a likely winner.

Funds for Pilot Studies in Basic POR

Finding funds for pilot studies is a serious obstacle for young, unproven investigators. Armed with new and challenging ideas, but lacking the data needed to support an RO1 grant application or an F32 fellowship application, they stand in desperate need of small sums with which to explore their hypotheses.

A most appropriate source of pilot study funds is the Biomedical Research Support Grant (BRSG), a mechanism that has served well for many years. This grant makes available to all institutions that receive NIH research funds an annual bloc grant for distribution within each institution to investigators with special financial needs. (The size of the BRSG grant to each institution is determined as a percentage of the amount of its total NIH research support.) A research dean in charge of the local distribution of BRSG funds can be extremely influential in recruiting young investigators into careers in clinical research by supporting their initial explorations.

Alternatively, the GCRC Branch itself could set up a BRSG-type mechanism, awarding each program director the discretionary use of a sum that represents a small percentage of the annual funding to his particular unit. Such a fund would enable each director and his Advisory Committee to support pilot studies in Basic POR by innovative young investigators under the supervision of sympathetic mentors.

A third source of pilot study money can sometimes be found in the NIH Center Core Grants (P30 grants) that support the specialized facilities required for categorical research across disciplinary lines. Devoting some of that funding to Basic POR pilot studies would create a valuable alliance between GCRCs and nearby Center Core laboratories.

Awards for Excellence in Basic POR

Supportive deans for clinical research should ask themselves whether the time is ripe for establishing a national award for excellence in Basic POR. No such prize exists today, even though prestigious awards for outstanding achievements in non-clinical research and Applied POR have been in place for years. (Indeed, the 1990 Nobel Prize in Medicine and Physiology is only the ninth award in 90 years that honored basic research discoveries made in whole human beings.) Such an award would appeal primarily to foundations or donors in the private sector. The Institute of Medicine would serve as the ideal vehicle for its selection. It has a far deeper interest in clinical research than does the National Academy of Sciences.

THOUGHTS FOR POR SCIENTISTS IN GCRCS

There are three major issues that deserve greater attention by program directors of GCRCs and their major users: greater emphasis on mentorship, enhancement of POR activities, and recognition of the educational role of the GCRC in that institution.

POR Mentors

The physician-scientists who use the facilities of their GCRCs are the best natural recruiters of young investigators into POR. As role models, they assist young people in their early studies and in the presentation of these studies orally and in writing. Their responsibilities do not end there. They must also help young investigators apply for fellowships and early career awards. Indeed, success in winning such awards depends heavily on the reputation and accomplishments of the mentor, as well as on the competence of the young applicant.

Recruitment into all forms of biomedical research must begin early, even during the college years. This is particularly true for POR; pre-medical students must be shown that the study of human beings is a rewarding career with many personal satisfactions. An ideal starting point in this early recruitment effort would be the participation of POR scientists of U.S. medical schools as teachers of college courses in *human* physiology. Who is better equipped to teach such courses than enthusiastic researchers who are themselves engaged in human physiological research and in human genetics? The setting up of such courses, the choice of a teaching site, the curriculum, the advisability of including a laboratory experience—these considerations fall outside the limits of this book, but the idea of encouraging pre-medical students to substitute a course in human physiology for one in general biology in order to meet admissions requirements has real merit.

At medical schools, POR mentors must feel obliged to "sell" POR to students from the first days of their first year. Demonstrations of onging studies in patients, presented in simple language, can show that the study of humans requires imagination and that the highest scientific standards must apply. First-year students, suddenly overwhelmed by exposure to facts (and more facts), must learn also that current medical knowledge, while extremely sophisticated, is replete with uncertainties, unanswered questions, and opportunities for important contributions by inquiring minds. They must be shown that POR can be just as basic as molecular biology and other strictly laboratory activities, provided that the right questions are asked and addressed by teams of MDs working hand-in-glove with PhDs, using appropriate modern technologies.

In the curricula of most U.S. medical schools, pre-clinical teachers have the first contacts with students. As a result, they are the first to identify the most curious and inquiring students and to lure them to their laboratories for extra-curricular laboratory research. POR workers must demand equal time. They must make known their own activities, interests, and challenges, and take the time to identify inquiring minds early; they must not wait until such students reach their clinical years. Informal discussion groups can be organized around POR topics; paid summer jobs can be made available and widely advertised; social contacts with energetic mentors will allow students to gain valuable guidance on career pathways. Deans for clinical research must take the lead in these early recruitment activities.

POR mentors, whether engaged in Basic or Applied POR, also can serve as useful advisors to graduates in their residency years and can help them in making career decisions. Subspecialty training can be much more than exposure to management methods and procedures if MD and PhD preceptors make it their business to address the scientific deficiencies of their residents and fellows. POR mentors can attract bright young investigators into POR by introducing them to the training opportunities offered by the NIH, such as the K11 Physician-Scientist award and the R29 FIRST award. Indeed, success in winning such awards depends heavily on mentors' having established their own scientific credibility. Their close association with PhD partners would demonstrate to peer review groups that training in POR can be just as sophisticated as training in the reductionist disciplines of non-clinical research.

To sum up, those who recognize the clinical challenges presented by their patients' illnesses and are prepared to take advantage of the facilities in their hospitals for research on such patients must be effective mentors as well as physician-scientists. They must demonstrate their mentorship as early as contacts with students can be arranged.

Enhancement of POR Quantity and Quality

Program directors of GCRCs and other POR leaders can enhance the quality of POR in their institutions—and its quantity—in a number of ways, all of which require time, imagination, and energy. The overwhelming majority of program directors of the 73 GCRCs surveyed in 1987–88 (Chapter 10) yearned for a *critical mass of intellectual activity* in their units—that is, for a large enough number of POR investigators interacting with each other and serving as exciting and instructive role models for younger researchers.

How have ingenious directors been able to seek out potential users and thus to reach a critical mass? It goes without saying that they must make widely known the capabilities of their facilities for performing high-grade research, with trained assistance and at no cost for bed and board and for many laboratory aids. Potential users must be sought out; it is fatal to wait for investigators to request these services on their own initiatives.

Some directors have made it a practice, at least once each year, to read the abstracts of all grants funded throughout their institutions, looking for awardees who can be persuaded to carry out some of their programs in their GCRC's. Others, as members of their IRBs and thus exposed to all the research applications that require human subjects or materials of human origin, have persuaded some of those applicants that their studies can be performed advantageously in the GCRC. Still others have organized monthly luncheon seminars for the discussion of ongoing research and for exchanging information on procedures and techniques. The lure is a free lunch, but the payoff is information exchange. Attendees at such seminars learn that experimental designs and laboratory techniques are often transportable from one program to another.

Enterprising directors have built intellectual and informational bridges to POR investigators throughout their institutions, and in the process have found that some types of Applied POR can be carried out in their GCRCs. These bridges help to create the critical mass of POR activity that justifies strong institutional support by deans and department chairmen, and it excites the interest of medical students and residents in POR as a career. Particularly fruitful areas in which to build such bridges are those interdisciplinary programs—like AIDS, cancer, hypertension, diabetes, and nutrition—in which success depends on building a critical mass of inquiring minds working in different ways toward common goals. These multidisciplinary programs, financed almost exclusively by the various NIH Institutes, have the further advantage of being broadly program-based rather than project-oriented. Moreover, the longer life span of program projects offers a measure of job security to young investigators that is elusive in times of fiscal constraints.

GCRCs as Educational Centers

Some GCRCs see themselves as educational centers, rather than simply as resources like animal centers in which to house animals for experimental purposes. This educational role can be played in a number of ways. An enterprising program director can take the lead in inviting a small number of students to spend a year-out in mid-course, especially if that GCRC has strong mentor teams of MDs and PhDs working with modern technologies. Educationally oriented GCRCs take maximum advantage of the CAP program, which funds 2 to 3 years' support of promising young investigators who are not yet qualified as independent researchers to apply for RO1 grants. Educational GCRCs are well equipped to organize courses for PhDs in human pathophysiology, like that described at Tufts by Arias (1989). "Broadened" PhDs become interested in the challenges of POR and effective as partners with MDs in its performance.

Even more challenging, an educational GCRC is the ideal site from which to launch an MD-PhD program directed specifically at careers in POR. Such an initiative would parallel today's MSTP program, which produces graduates who pursue careers mainly in bench research. The organizational aspects of such a double-degree program can be no better managed in U.S. medical schools than by an imaginative GCRC director working in concert with a strong Advisory Committee; its success will depend on partnerships between MDs and PhDs that ensure a broad base of training in scientific design and modern technologies. Indeed, such partnerships could kindle the interest of a small number of highly selected college students in bedside research, perhaps catalyzed by a college course in human physiology taught by members of such teams.

Action at the National Level

GCRC directors and major users of POR facilities must occasionally leave their ivory towers and conspire to play a more visible political role.

First, they are in the best position to persuade talented POR colleagues nation-wide to join the NIH peer review process, from which many have fled in recent years. By volunteering to accept this responsibility, they will help to ensure the survival of POR while performing an important public service. The IRGs of the various Institutes are likely to be most receptive to such advances. The Institutes, through their administrators for extramural research, are more interested in the prosperity of clinical research of all kinds than are the administrators of the DRG. Indeed, the Institutes' IRGs are made up of more senior extramural experts who are likely to be sympathetic to the development of re-search talent and not simply to the production of research data.

Second, POR researchers are ideally qualified to be chosen as extramural advisors to the various Institutes for review of bedside research in the NIH Clinical Center, a process that now is totally internal and woefully inadequate. If the NIH can be prodded to set up these urgently needed external reviews, POR researchers must certainly volunteer to serve.

Third, POR researchers are admirably prepared to remedy the crying need for teaching aids and instructional materials with which to introduce young investigators to the integrative discipline of POR. Today there are no manuals or textbooks for POR, as there are for biochemistry, molecular biology, and other reductionist disciplines; this is a serious limitation to the future health of POR. Two sorts of instructional aids are needed:

1. *Experimental design* can advantageously be taught by MD mentors, who can analyze with their young researchers the published reports of previous years that have led to new understandings of human physiology and disease. Design is a critical element in experimental work that does not become outmoded with the passage of time, as do experimental techniques.
2. *Modern technologies* that must be applied in POR can be effectively taught by PhDs with years of experience in new techniques. (The value of this practice has been proved in the 2-year instruction program of postgraduate MDs by PhDs at the Department of Medicine in Pittsburgh (Lehotay et al., 1982).

Thus, MDs who are expert in POR are qualified to instruct their apprentices in matters of experimental design, as are their PhD partners in matters of modern technologies. But it is not textbooks or manuals that are needed in this era of computer-assisted education. Rather, it is videotapes and discs prepared by experts in the advertising and TV industries, working hand-in-hand with the country's most articulate and knowledgeable POR experts. Learning can occur in real time at terminals through nationwide networking or by means of hard copy (even in color). Certain subjects lend themselves to animation, others to user-interactive question-and-answer formats. POR is a wide open field for educational innovation; that time has arrived!

In the future, it is conceivable that POR will not die but flourish, and that annual meetings will once again be organized on a national scale in which a broad spectrum of research results will be presented to audiences of POR investigators and their apprentices. I sense a considerable longing among physician-scientists for the stimulation of hearing about the accomplishments of POR researchers in disciplines outside their own, and for the personal satisfactions that characterized the meetings of generalists in earlier decades. While it is certain that specialized symposia will multiply in number and in the complexity of their subject matter, there will be a return, I believe, to generalism in medical research as the need for integration of the discoveries of reductionists is recognized. Indeed, a *Journal of POR* is not beyond conception, filling a role that has been abandoned by the *Journal of Experimental Medicine* and by the *Journal of Clinical Investigation.*

SUMMARY AND CONCLUSIONS

The special endangerment of Basic POR cannot be overcome *in the long term* if the serious defects underlying American medicine as a whole fail to be resolved. The primary mission of U.S. medical schools—namely, medical education—has been dwarfed by the dominance there of research since the 1950s and of service to patients for the sake of income generation since the 1970's. The first is a reflection of a sudden inflow of research dollars from the federal government; the second, of the impact of the Medicare/Medicaid legislation of 1965 on medical economics. The only solutions that I can see for the future health of medical education are to separate as much as possible the teaching-research function from the service function in U.S. academic health centers and to reduce the number of MDs graduated each year. Then, in schools scaled down in size and streamlined in costs, we must seek a better balance between teaching and research in which each professional group is rewarded fully and appropriately for its special skills.

However it is attained, collegiality among medical school faculties must be re-established for the sake of students, faculties, and patients. The purposes: protected time for more inspired teaching and cultivation of a spirit of inquiry, distinct from rote learning; protected time for a smaller number of more highly qualified researchers working in all phases of clinical research; and the opportunity for faculties to re-assess their values in regard to reward systems and the reduction of barriers between MDs and PhDs.

To the leaders in U.S. medical schools, attention is called to the special advantages of establishing associate deans for clinical research and to the crying need for strong institutional support for Basic POR scientists.

To POR scientists in GCRCs, attention is called to the need for stronger and more innovative mentorship; to means by which a critical mass of intellectual endeavor and excitement can be achieved at POR sites; to the value of creating an educational environment in their GCRCs, as distinct from a mere service function, in which MD-PhD programs can be organized for training young people in integrative research; and to the need for training aids in POR (which are totally lacking today) that capitalize on modern computer- and video-assisted technical skills.

15

Need for New Strategies and Balances at the NIH

Blame for the endangerment of Basic POR cannot be laid entirely on the doorstep of U.S. medical education. Policies at the NIH are equally if not more determinative in righting the imbalances in biomedical research that now threaten the survival of Basic POR. This chapter is addressed to the five elements of NIH that can play it safe by holding tight to the status quo—or can venture to experiment with new strategies: the Director's Office, the 13 Institutes, the Clinical Center, the GCRC Branch, and the DRG.

THOUGHTS FOR THE DIRECTOR'S OFFICES

The post–World War II growth and development of the NIH occurred during a period in U.S. biomedicine characterized by enthusiasm, optimism, innovation, experimentation, and a missionary spirit of helpfulness to scientists "beyond the Beltway" on the part of those in administrative positions in Bethesda. These qualities, backed up by seemingly limitless federal funds, made the NIH the envy of the biomedical world and a model for change in other countries.

The consequences of becoming dependent on NIH funding were rarely questioned. Universities and academic medical centers were delighted to receive generous funding to expand and modernize, with the result that medical schools grew in number from 70 to more than 120, medical school enrollments doubled, faculty numbers quadrupled, and medical centers extended their reach and consequently their responsibilities far beyond the 1910 Flexner model of a modest medical educational system steeped in an atmosphere of intellectual curiosity and inquiry.

The NIH itself burgeoned in acreage, buildings, administrative staff, and outreach, and its intramural scientific staff grew in number even more rapidly than the space available for it. President Richard Nixon's War on Cancer was the wedge that split a unified NIH administration into many categorical Institutes in 1972, each with its own mission and administrative structure to further that mission, so that in the last 20 years the NIH has become a colossus. Its scientists as well as its administration deserve the admiration it receives worldwide, but inevitably there comes a time to take stock, even of colossi, and I believe that time has arrived. I intend no irreverence when I question whether the current period in U.S. biomedicine is still one of enthusiasm, optimism, innovativeness, and experimentation, and whether the missionary spirit of unselfish service to others still prevails in the extramural roles of the NIH.

Before proceeding to an analysis of the relationships within the NIH internal staff and of its extramural offices to their beneficiaries, I want to address the Director's Office about three general concerns because they are matters of importance for the NIH as a whole. They deal with the need to establish better mechanisms for evaluating the present and future performance of the many intra- and extramural programs of the NIH; the desirability of concentrating more on the development of scientifically talented people and less on protocol-driven research; and the necessity to provide more effective support for bedside research without lessening its support for bench research.

Accountability

Reviewing the performance of the various components and functions of NIH can no longer be left to intramural staff; the internal reviews of past years have all too often reeked of turf protection. Background reports performed by paid outside contractors—consultants who are not themselves biomedical scientists—can be useful in assembling the necessary facts and figures. But judgments based on those data are far more likely to be analytical, constructive, and innovative if they are made by extramural experts, openly and at regular intervals and with assured continuity in decision making.

The NIH complains that outside experts are increasingly unwilling to serve as NIH reviewers and study section members. This situation could change if the individuals invited to take part in these time-consuming and arduous tasks were persuaded that their efforts were being taken seriously, and that some sort of feedback to their suggestions and responses were set up and given continuity by avoidance of one-time ad hoc meetings. Such reviewers should meet at least annually and serve 3- to 4-year staggered terms. The present system of assembling ad hoc groups for single meetings on policy matters, with or without written responses by the components being reviewed, fails to provide feedback and follow-up and is little better than tokenism.

Training vs. Research Results (People vs. Projects)

Peer reviewers of applications for traditional investigator-initiated research projects have tended more and more to judge the merit of such applications on the basis of the likelihood of obtaining valid experimental data, and less on the originality and inventiveness of the proposals. Faced with fiscal constraints, applicants consider rigidly standardized protocols to be the safest way to design an acceptable application. How can the right balance be achieved between the development of innovative scientists (through the funding of training grants, fellowships, and start-up grants) and the accumulation of new data (through traditional research projects)?

The NIH is continuously faced with this balancing act. Everyone agrees that well-trained investigators will inevitably produce good science, but it is far easier to pass judgment on the details of risk-evasive proposals than to assess the quality of the talents of young investigators, many of whom have not yet established a track record in research. A committee of the IOM chaired by Floyd Bloom addressed this serious issue in its 1990 report—"A Strategy to Restore Balance." By recommending that training-grant monies be increased by 60% over the next 10 years at the expense of funds for traditional research projects, this committee showed its concern for the development of young scientists.

Laboratory Science and Clinical Research

The widely held prejudice that laboratory work is science, and that clinical research is not, is rooted positively in the power of modern technologies that are ever more sensitive, qualitatively and quantitatively, and negatively in the lack of controls that make research on human beings so difficult. Nevertheless, bedside research can be as basic as bench research; it is the nature of the questions asked that determine their basic-ness. Given the choice between the power of new technologic approaches and the difficulties encountered in performing truly basic clinical research, young research-minded MDs have leaned increasingly toward reductionist research. It is more precise and controllable and, accordingly, more likely to win in the RO1 scramble.

The argument has been made in previous chapters that clinical research is composed of several different activities, some reductionistic and others integrative in nature; and that these two intellectual disciplines, while fundamentally different, are complementary and both deserving of full support. Yet the pace of progress in reaching new understandings of human biology through these two disciplines is very different, and this difference in pace demands that separate yardsticks be used in measuring their movement.

The NIH and its reviewing bodies appear to have taken the view that major attention will be paid to whatever discipline seems to be producing the most provocative data most rapidly. But the NIH could have adopted the longer-term view that, since both approaches are essential to medical progress, both must be adequately supported, however different their paces. The biomedical world is now in a reductionist mood, and it takes justifiable pride in the recent advances achieved in molecular biology. But it would seem obvious that, after the parts of a whole organism have been completely disassembled, they must be put back together in such a way that the reassembled organism is identical in form and function to the original. It is the integrationists who must devise ways to ensure that the original whole and the re-assembled whole are identical; and, if not, to explain why not. Someone has reminded us that it is more difficult to put a pocket watch back together again than to take it to pieces.

The gatekeepers of extramural funding, the IRGs of the Institutes and the

DRG, are responsible for achieving an effective balance between reductionistic and integrative research, with an eye to the future as well as the present. The record shows that this balance has gone awry. Research on human beings is falling dangerously behind non-clinical research in the awarding decisions of the IRGs, and the most integrative activity of clinical research (namely, Basic POR) is the hardest hit of all. The NIH can perform a powerful service by advertising its understanding of this imbalance and by taking appropriate steps (see below) to correct the imbalances and inequities.

THOUGHTS FOR THE VARIOUS INSTITUTES

The missions of the disease-oriented NIH Institutes have led them to support clinical research more strongly than does the DRG and the NIGMS, as evidenced by their emphasis on program project grants, centers, and fellowships.

Targeted Funding

For this reason, I would point out that a powerfully encouraging signal to physician-scientists interested in exploring basic questions in human biology would be the decision by one or more Institutes to allocate a designated percentage of their total appropriations to the support of Basic POR. I recognize that earmarking funds for a specific purpose sets a dangerous precedent; nevertheless, *at this time* a decision of this kind has real merit. It would indicate that those Institutes do not intend to let Basic POR wither away; that its practitioners, now in short supply and rapidly disappearing, should be quickly replaced through vigorous recruitment tactics; and that measures should be taken to guarantee that Basic POR is pursued by scientists who are well-equipped with modern technologic tools and skills. *The dedication of funds to Basic POR has the merit of making it possible for POR applications to compete for funding against each other,* instead of competing against dissimilar applications for non-clinical research, as at present.

Decisions for targeted funding are not without precedent. The Human Genome Project is such a case; AIDS research is another. Both are justified on the basis of their importance for the future. In the first case, gene research promises to enlarge our understanding of human biology; in the second, the health hazards of AIDS and the biological novelty of that disease process are unprecedented. Targeted funding for Basic POR is important for the future prosperity of all clinical research.

Large Controlled Trials

The several Institutes, by dint of their disease orientation, are primary supporters of large-scale, controlled clinical trials of new drugs, procedures, and devices. Such trials are immensely expensive in dollars and in human effort, yet it is absolutely essential that they be undertaken to ensure the safety and efficacy of the agent under test. Whether to mount such trials at the NIH Clinical Center, or in GCRCs, or even in extramural research-intensive medical institutions—those are decisions that merit very careful re-thinking.

Such trials demand clinical observational skills and fastidious quality control measures of many sorts, but once the experimental design of a trial has been drawn up, the protocol cannot be altered until the trial is finished. Why not perform such trials in institutional settings that are expert in the delivery of medical services to large populations of patients and put them under the control of MDs who are primarily clinicians, rather than educators and researchers? For the Institutes to perform such trials at the Clinical Center, which was *established as an institution in which to carry out experimental studies in human subjects that cannot be done elsewhere,* is justified only when better understanding of a procedure's mode of action might lead to deeper biological insights and to applications other than those originally intended. The unique mission of the Clinical Center, with its extraordinarily ample facilities, makes it an inappropriate site for those controlled trials that can equally well be performed in research-non-intensive sites. The various Institutes should dedicate their clinical facilities to Basic POR, not Applied POR.

THOUGHTS FOR THE CLINICAL CENTER

The Clinical Center at the NIH can and should be the standard setter for Basic POR throughout the world and the role model for GCRCs in U.S. medical schools. That is not the case today, even though the Clinical Center is the most richly funded research hospital in the land. It can attract patients for study from any part of the United States and is empowered to pay their travel expenses to and from Bethesda; in addition, its physician-scientists gain precious time for research by not having to compete for funding of their studies with extramural POR investigators.

There has never been a systematic exchange of research information or of research physicians between the very large Clinical Center and the much smaller GCRCs in U.S. medical schools. Intra- and extramural physicians know very little about each other's activities, challenges, and problems except through the research literature and through informal meetings at national conferences. In the face of this communication gap, how can high-quality role modeling be demonstrated and uniformly high standards set and met?

In addition, there have been no systematic, perceptive reviews of the scientific merit of bedside research at the Clinical Center, except internally, and no attempt to compare those programs with others carried out in U.S. medical schools or in the 74 GCRCs. The one and only complete review of Clinical Center activities, chaired by D.W. Seldin and reported in 1985, devoted only two pages to the protocols of its in-patient studies. Eight extramural POR experts concluded after a "paper review" of 50 protocols on bedside research that "there was substantial variation in the quality of the protocols reviewed, from truly outstanding to quite poor . . . some proposals would not pass the scrutiny of the extramural peer review process."

The boards of scientific counselors of the various Institutes are responsible for periodic reviews of their bedside research, but they have neither the time nor the expertise to undertake such audits in depth. The need for frequent periodic reviews by extramural POR experts is clearly evident. Those reviews should be carried out by external review teams reporting to each Institute before, during, and after such studies are performed in the beds allocated to each, and should meet periodically and not on an ad hoc basis. An ongoing review process would be instructive as well as morale-building for intramural physicians who are engaged in bedside research, and such review groups would serve as advocates to those scientific directors who are inclined to allocate their funds to bench research rather than to bedside studies. The process would also serve to bring intra- and extramural POR investigators together scientifically in ways no longer afforded by national meetings of clinical investigators.

Fiscal constraints on the Clinical Center (see Chapter 10) are increasingly limiting the amount of bedside research. This phenomenon can be explained by the fact that the Center is funded each year, not directly by a congressional appropriation but by payments to the Center by each Institute. The size of each of those levies is based on each Institute's bed allocation, bed usage, and ancillary costs for special services (pathology, surgery, CT scans, etc.), and those patient costs have been rising steadily.

Increasing costs of POR at the Clinical Center can be met by the Institutes' scientific directors in only two ways—by devoting more of the funds allocated for non-clinical laboratory research to bedside research or by reducing the amount of POR pursued by their clinical scientists. Those scientific directors who lean toward undiminished funding of laboratory research in their Institutes discourage the performance of bedside research in the Clinical Center, and as bed usage decreases, bed costs increase still further. This vicious cycle will kill the Clinical Center.

Counterproductive competition for funds in each Institute can be avoided if Congress is persuaded to give the Center its own budget allocation, separate from those of the individual Institutes. In this event, the Center would be in a position to offer its clinical services to each of the Institutes *at no charge*. The Center would be obligated to keep track of all of its patient costs in great detail and thus would be prepared annually to defend those expenditures to Congress, as well as to justify the next year's budgetary request. The cost to the taxpayer would be neither greater nor less than it is now, since the current $200 million annual expenditure at the Clinical Center would be derived directly from Congress, rather than indirectly from the several Institutes. The bedside researchers of the several Institutes would compete with each other for bed space on the merits of their research programs, and would not compete for funds with their colleagues in purely laboratory research. Consequently, the present unequal competition for intramural funds would cease, and the scientific directors would be relieved of some vexing budgetary decisions. They would still be directly responsible for the quality of the bedside research in their Institutes, and should share this responsibility with extramural reviewing teams assembled for assistance in this judgment.

This recommendation for change in fiscal policy raises a companion question: should intra- and extramural Basic POR activities be merged by creating a single agency for POR, the scope of which would be nation-wide? With headquarters in Bethesda, such as agency would represent the bringing together of two small armies of physician-scientists into a single enterprise with common goals. It would ensure the informational exchange on POR that now is lacking, as well as exchanges of POR scholars. It would lead to the setting of a single high standard of quality for POR throughout the country. It would benefit by having a single cadre of administrators. Such a consolidation would remove the GCRC function from the DRR, where it is inherently a misfit. GCRC's are not just resources; they should be educational centers, as well as centers of excellence in basic POR.

Simply merging the Clinical Center with the GCRC system would create an agency spending $300 million annually in current dollars—4% of the total NIH appropriation in 1991, with no increase in costs to the taxpayer. This recommendation certainly deserves careful study.

THOUGHTS FOR THE GCRC BRANCH

Aside from the question just raised (a single national agency for POR), the branch is faced with a number of compelling problems that can be addressed prior to such a merger. The problems are soluble.

Shifting Funds

The current GCRC appropriation, now approaching $130 million annually, is unlikely to grow larger in the near future, yet there are a number of demands on these funds that must be met if POR is to prosper in the several sites in which these special centers are now located:

1. If program directors of the highest caliber are to be attracted and held in these key positions, they must be fully salaried and not dependent on income derived from private practice.
2. Each program director must be supported by middle-level, fully salaried POR investigators. Researchers in middle-level ranks are essential role models for younger investigators, and their presence on GCRC units will help to achieve a critical mass of intellectual activity.
3. Program directors need allocations of discretionary funds that can be devoted to the support of the pilot studies of young investigators not yet qualified to apply for an independent grant.

If these demands on the Branch are considered to be important, and if the total GCRC appropriation is unlikely to increase, can the Branch justify its continuing to fund 74 GCRCs? The answer seems obvious: the difficult decision to close down one or more such units must be faced if the program as a whole is to be protected. Such an action is not without precedent; 93 centers in 1970 were reduced to 75 in 1980.

Promoting the CAP Program

The GCRC Branch has an educational job to do in persuading its various program directors to take greater advantage of the CAP program, which on a competitive basis offers salaries and some expense money to as many as two young POR investigators per center for as long as 2 years each. That program currently costs the Branch 2–3% of its annual appropriation. In view of the need to bring more young scholars into POR, an increase in this proportion should be voted by its GCRC Advisory Committee and funded by reducing the total number of Centers.

All of these recommendations will cost money; this can be accomplished only by scaling down the number of units now funded, since an increase in congressional appropriations for the Branch seems unlikely. The wisdom of consolidating the Branch with the NIH Clinical Center into a single agency for POR becomes even more compelling, and to Congress more persuasive: one purpose, one agency, one administration, one appropriation.

THOUGHTS FOR THE DRG

Winning an RO1 grant is today the single most important determinant of a successful career in biomedical research by MD and PhD researchers, and the DRG is by all odds the major gatekeeper. It is no longer justifiable to leave the initial and almost always decisive judgments on RO1 applications for POR in the hands of study sections that are increasingly unsympathetic to such applications and increasingly unprepared to judge them.

Study Section Reforms

The management of the DRG seems determined not to concern itself with the waning fortunes of Basic POR and seems not to realize that integrative research as well as reductionistic research must be supported. The following courses of action can work to achieve that balance so as to ensure the long-term prosperity of biomedical research on which medical progress and the public's health depend:

1. Invite POR-competent scientists to become members of study sections to which POR applications are assigned, and beware of the dominance in these sections of MDs who are chiefly molecular biologists.

2. Re-think today's almost exclusive reliance on the perceived worthiness of research protocols that in times of financial distress inevitably become risk-aversive, more pedestrian, more conservative, more safe, and less innovative. If investigators have established a track record in their research, let this weigh much more heavily in making awards. If track records have not yet been achieved, reward the most innovative, risk-taking proposal.

3. *Most* important, make a clean break with the past by establishing study sections dedicated exclusively to consideration of Basic POR applications. Can this action be justified without being labeled special pleading? The questions that can be addressed in humans are different from those that are directed to molecules or subcellular particles or animals, and investigators who have learned to frame those different kinds of questions do so in very different ways. Because physicists think and act differently from chemists, and physiologists from microbiologists, the NIH has wisely devised mechanisms by which the research proposals in a given specialty are reviewed by practitioners of that discipline. Thus, there have come to be study sections in microbiology, pathology, pharmacology, physiology, and many other biomedical disciplines. Accordingly, because Basic POR is an integrative discipline, distinctly different in many ways from the reductionist disciplines, there are compelling reasons for the review of POR proposals by experts in POR.

I submit that an important determinant of the declining success rate of Basic POR applications is the lack of appreciation by reductionists (and especially by MDs who have become molecular biologists) of the restraints imposed on POR by such practical matters as patient availability, by ethical considerations, and by the heterogeneity among human subjects that at one and the same time is a burden and a hallmark of human experimentation.

Accordingly, I urge that Basic POR applications be reviewed and evaluated by study sections made up of members who have themselves carried out meaningful studies in humans, who understand the restraints under which POR studies must be performed, who are sympathetic to the goals of POR, and who have learned through experience to recognize the incredible opportunities afforded by experiments of nature (that is, disease) for gaining new insights into human biology.

The argument has been raised that a Basic POR study section could not effectively review the various kinds of POR applications coming out of the many different subspecialties of medicine. Consideration of the current array of more than 100 study sections invalidates that argument. Each one is served by such a wide array of subspecialists with disparate skills that there is almost no common language among them. It is no wonder that any given POR application fares badly today when thrown into gatherings of such diverse talents.

This recommendation is in no way a plea for less rigorous scientific reviews of Basic POR applications. The percentiling system now employed by the various Institutes for relating the award decisions of the many DRG study sections to each other ensures that only the best applications passing through each of the study sections will be funded; and percentiling will apply to a POR study section's deliberations just as it does to the recommendations of other study sections. Thus, if a given Institute's payline allows only 15% of all approved applications to be funded in that year, then only 15% of the approved POR applications will be so awarded. In essence, this policy change will *ensure that basic POR applications are rated against each other,* and not, as at present, against those filed by non-clinical researchers or by clinical researchers pursuing reductionistic goals.

Changes in Grant Application Forms

For many years, the application forms for NIH grants requested that co-PIs be specifically named. The NSF continues to request this information, but the NIH abandoned the practice for purely administrative reasons in 1981. To promote the advantages of partnerships of MDs and PhDs in clinical research, the practice of listing PIs and co-PIs should be reinstituted. This is recommended, not simply in fairness to the aspirations and skills of co-PI's, but more importantly, in order to allow the DRG to follow more precisely the careers of its major recipients, many of whose names are now lost to the DRG's IMPAC database.

In addition, it would be extremely informative for applicants on NIH grants to indicate the intention of their proposals as either Non-Clinical or as one of the Seven Categories of Clinical Research that I have shown to be useful in describing the several meanings of that term. This information, added to the DRG's CRISP database, would allow the NIH to follow time trends in the research activities of its applicants and awardees. It would also be useful in reporting its annual expenditures for various kinds of research and training to Congress, as well as to those offices of the NIH administration that are responsible for achieving an optimal balance between training goals and research results.

Is it of any use to attempt to improve the study section system of review when funds are now so limited that fewer than 25% of study section–approved applications are funded? The only answer to this question is that *times do change.* We must act on the premise that the research environment will eventually improve, and when it does, the most equitable and farsighted systems must be in place, ready to take hold and perform wisely.

SUMMARY AND CONCLUSIONS

Stronger institutional support for POR in U.S. medical schools will not, by itself, ensure that POR regains its proper place in the broad arena of clinical research. The NIH must take responsibility for a complementary role in reaching this objective. To that end, it must consider new strategies for addressing the many concerns that have emerged over the last 25 years in its own intramural operation and in its relations with extramural partners in biomedical research. The NIH is no longer setting the pace in clinical research nationally, or in POR in particular, even though it controls the major share of financial support for those activities. It can reassert this leadership if it gives serious consideration to righting the imbalances that have come to exist in its backing of non-clinical and clinical research extramurally and intramurally.

To the NIH director, attention is called to the urgent need for more effective extramural evaluations of all intramural activities, and especially of the bedside research at the Clinical Center; to the eminent desirability of concentrating more on the development of scientific talent and less on protocol-driven research; and to the need to enunciate the understanding of the NIH that the current imbalances between reductionist and integrative research disciplines will be reduced.

To the directors of the various NIH Institutes and of the Clinical Center, attention is called to the immediate need to set aside funds for training and grants in Basic POR; to the essentiality of committing their bedside research facilities to experimental studies in human subjects that cannot be done elsewhere in the United States; to the eminent wisdom of creating extramural panels to review the quality of the bedside research of each Institute in the Clinical Center; to the advantages of furnishing all Clinical Center resources free of charge to each of the Institutes by pressing Congress for a separate budget line item in support of the Center; and to the wisdom of creating a single agency in charge of POR at the Clinical Center and at all GCRCs.

To the GCRC Branch, attention is called to the economic necessity of reducing the current number of GCRCs in order to obtain funds for full-salary support of all program directors and middle-level POR investigators at the most productive units, and for pilot studies by young investigators at the various GCRCs.

To the DRG, attention is called to the need for a number of re-structurings in its present study sections: more MD members with personal experience in POR and fewer who are out-and-out reductionists, and a stronger focus on innovative research and less on strictly protocolized projects. Above all, attention is called to the essentiality of establishing one or more new study sections for review of POR applications by experts with personal experience in POR, in recognition that POR is an integrative discipline different in its objectives, pace, style, and management from the reductionist disciplines.

16

An Agenda for Change

CONCERNS FOR CLINICAL RESEARCH AND
FOR MEDICAL EDUCATION

The vagaries of clinical research are deeply concerning to its practitioners, both MDs and PhDs, who consider that their careers are seriously threatened by the current shortage of funds for research. Even worse, the insecurities of established researchers seem frightening to their younger colleagues, many of whom are turning away from research careers in favor of more secure futures elsewhere. Even though market forces will eventually create a new balance between the supply of and demand for biomedical scientists, in the long term it is the public that will pay the highest price for these damages, because medical progress depends directly on the well-being of an active scientific work force. At this moment, however, the public is far more troubled by rising health care costs than by the viability of the biomedical research establishment.

Likewise, the majority of U.S. physicians have serious but far different concerns of their own. Some 90% of the active physicians in the United States are engaged in medical practice. Their attention is appropriately focused on the diagnosis and treatment of illness, and, better yet, its prevention and the preservation of health. Not personally engaged in the development of new methods of diagnosis and treatment but in their applications, they are obliged by the public's expectations to take full advantage of these advances, despite their increasing costliness and relative inaccessibility. But they are increasingly irritated by the rash of regulations imposed on them by layers of governmental agencies requesting laborious accountings for these practices. And so it is not to this large segment of the American MD work force that we can look for solutions to the dilemmas of clinical research.

Threatened researchers must look instead to American medical schools for relief, for the dilemmas in clinical research stem in large part from the failure of these schools to hew to their primary mission as educational institutions. Attention to teaching was eclipsed first by distracting fixations on research when research funding was abundant in the 1950s and 1960s, and then, after 1965, by the economic burdens imposed on them by the escalating costs of health care. To overcome these burdens, the clinical departments have grown in size, completely out of proportion to the number of medical students, and income generation has taken the place of both research and teaching as the major activity of the full-time clinical faculties. Even so, productivity in research is still the yard-stick by which priorities, tenure, and prizes are measured; a genius for teaching is only grudgingly rewarded. As medical schools have become more and more curriculum-driven, contacts between students and faculty have become less and less stimulating. Collegiality among overspecialized faculties also has been eroded.

Among researchers, short-term objectives have taken the place of long-term goals, and risk-taking explorations of puzzling research questions have given way to sure-fire "projects" as the keys to professional advancement and security. These and other considerations have led physician-scientists away from Basic POR, which is difficult, time-consuming, costly, and often uncertain in out-come. Over the last two decades, the reductionism of molecular biology, with its stripping away of variables, has largely replaced the integrative research that is typical of Basic POR. Thus, a major imbalance in clinical research now exists; and this imbalance has been left untended by those medical school authorities whose focus on income generation has driven them toward a growing dependence on medical service to patients in ever-larger health centers and on outside grant support for research that is increasingly reductionistic.

The NIH is now the "keeper" of these imbalances in clinical research, not through intention but rather through inattention. This "greatest social achieve-ment of the twentieth century," to paraphrase Lewis Thomas, has become top-heavy, authoritarian, and unresponsive. The layers of management at NIH are almost impenetrable for those outside the NIH, and even for insiders. The status quo at NIH is inviolate, and turf protection is the name of the game at all ranks.

PROSPECTS FOR SOLUTIONS

Resolving the dilemmas in clinical research must be approached from two direc-tions simultaneously. First, a clearer understanding of the essentially of integra-tive research must be sought at all levels—among medical students and their faculties, as well as by funding organizations (public and private). Potential re-searchers must be shown that the pursuit of integrative research on whole organ-isms is highly satisfying as a career, as well as essential for medical progress.

Second, an environment in which integrative research is admired, respected, and rewarded must be created at the same time as its essentiality is recognized. Medical schools certainly cannot and will not turn away from reductionistic re-search; rather, they must set up a POR-friendly atmosphere alongside it. This can occur only through fundamental changes in reward systems, in which pro-motions are based on comparisons made *within* specific categories of faculty members and not *across* those categorical boundaries. These changes can take place only if NIH revamps its peer review system in such a way that the merits of Basic POR proposals are judged in competition with each other, and not in competition with the many different disciplines of reductionism. NIH must demonstrate its recognition that the development of talent is more important than the harvesting of research results: the latter is inevitable if the former is ensured.

My personal agenda for change has four specifics:

1. The atmosphere in U.S. medical schools must be made more intimate and collegial. The larger the incoming class of students, the less possible it is to abandon didactic teaching and rote learning. It is heartening to learn that a half dozen or more U.S. schools have recently undertaken radically new educational efforts in which small groups of students meet almost daily in the pre-clinical years with carefully chosen tutors. The goal of this educational departure is to encourage problem-solving rather than mastery of factual information, and to do so through student interactions and explorations of the literature that are guided only when necessary by the tutor. These intimate contacts with individual faculty members have re-kindled a spirit of inquiry and collegiality that cannot thrive when the curriculum is dominated by days full of lectures by a parade of faculty members who rarely have personal contacts with their audiences.

For example, at Harvard Medical School, the incoming class of 175 matriculants is divided into five equal parts (called "societies"). Thus, in its pre-clinical years, Harvard is no longer one but five schools, each rather independent of the others. Each of those societies is subdivided into small units of six to eight students who meet with a single faculty member three mornings a week to explore problems in clinical medicine. The essence of this "New Pathway," begun in 1984, is the interactions of small groups of students who teach each other how to recognize the many faces of medical problems and to reach solutions by understanding the origins of those problems. This newly constituted teaching faculty has found these exercises to be highly rewarding educational experiences for themselves. Once the novelty of this new curriculum wears off, the high cost of faculty time (3 to 4 consecutive months for each mentor) will be accepted by them if good teaching is appropriately rewarded.

2. Medical schools must find ways to divorce themselves from their dependence on income generation through provision of medical services to the general community. If the education of students once again becomes their main reason for being, and if that objective is better achieved by admitting smaller incoming classes (or fragmented classes, as at Harvard), then the costs for faculty salaries, meeting rooms, laboratories, in-patient teaching beds, and out-patient teaching clinics will be greatly reduced. Needless to say, the needs of the community for general medical attention must still be met, but this should no longer be the responsibility of the schools, but rather that of the medical centers whose primary goal is service, not teaching. Today's conflicting demands on full-time faculty members for service, research, *and* teaching can no longer be justified by the economics of service-generated income.

3. Centers for clinical research within these schools must assume the role of educational centers in addition to serving as facilities for performance of Basic POR. They will need the strong institutional support that can best be provided though the appointment of deans for clinical research who are themselves researchers. The largest site for clinical research in the United States, the Clinical

Center at the NIH, must become the standard setter that it is not today. This can be accomplished if the Clinical Center is awarded its own budget by Congress, separate from the budgets of the 13 Institutes, and if Basic POR becomes dominant at that site. A single agency for POR should be created in which the activities of the NIH Clinical Center are loosely coordinated with those of the smaller GCRCs that are now located in the more research-intensive medical schools throughout the United States. This will have many advantages aside from greater efficiency and economy: the morale and enthusiasm of physician-scientists for Basic POR will be raised; the recruitment of potential POR scientists will become easier; and the benefits of working partnerships between MDs and PhDs will be more easily demonstrated.

4. Finally, we must face up to what I have called the Malthusian dilemma in biomedical research. We are currently "breeding" more scientists than the public and private systems can support. MD and PhD researchers, be they clinical or non-clinical in their research orientation, have been reproducing themselves at a rate that has become alarming. If the most talented scientists are to be brought into and held in research careers, at what stage would "birth control" be least detrimental?

I would opt for making the critical choices among research-minded individuals only after each has been given a reasonable opportunity to demonstrate his own measure of imaginativeness, innovativeness, motivation, courage, and persistence. For MDs, I would offer training and early career support to all who feel they want to test their strengths in the research world, preferably after 2 to 3 years of hospital experience. I would ensure each of them at least 8 years of continuous support, free from the harassment of serial grant applications. At the end of that period, I would expect some Solomonic mechanism of highly selective peer review to pick out those researchers who have proved themselves most worthy of continued support in long-term research careers. Those passed over will move into teaching, or into practice, or into some other medical activity, and with some anguish, but they will have had a fair chance to prove their mettle. Those who win continued research support—the research mentors of tomorrow—will be considerably fewer in number than our presently aging biomedical research population and more productive, and their replicands necessarily fewer in number. As this Malthusian dilemma is aborted, high-quality research will nevertheless be ensured.

To set up barriers at a much earlier stage—for instance, at the end of residency training—would eliminate late bloomers and favor those who concentrate in college and at medical school on science over those with a more general educational background. This process would lead to an undesirably narrow range of talents among the research community and to another kind of specialization that would undermine the collegiality of the faculties of these sites.

However it is accomplished, something must be done about the overproduction of biomedical scientists. It must be done in a way that is fair to all, and is most productive of a smaller group of highly talented, middle-aged researchers serving as inspiring mentors for the young hopefuls following them.

L'ENVOI

In examining the future prospects of clinical research in the United States, I have asked whether POR is essential for reaching deeper understandings of human biology and for bringing better health to the people of this country. And from the outset, I have weighed the proposition that the new technologies of molecular biology can be relied on to solve the medical problems of the future. I have rejected the proposition that POR can be abandoned.

It is my deeply held conviction that *all* forms of biomedical research (including POR) must be urgently pursued, because all are complementary and none trivial. Nevertheless, it is clear that Basic POR is in greatest jeopardy today, and in need of much stronger support by institutional forces in U.S. medical schools and by the NIH than it now receives.

I can ask no more of the readers of this book than that they take these warning signals seriously and be willing to debate the pros and cons of the remedies I have offered. I hope that the correction of current imbalances will take place more rapidly than simply through evolution. Solutions will be found if the issues are clearly recognized and openly debated.

References

The following reference list represents only those items referred to in the text of this book. A more complete reference list, dealing with many aspects of clinical research since Beaumont in the 1820s, medical education, and U.S. academic health centers, and consisting of more than 150 pages of annotated bibliography, is available on request to the author at a cost to cover mailing and reproduction ($10).

AAHC Directory 1989. Washington, DC, Association of American Health Centers, 1989.

AAMC Data Book. Washington, DC, Association of American Medical Colleges. 1990.

AAMC Faculty Roster System: Numbers Book. Washington, DC, Association of American Medical Colleges, 1988.

AAMC Institutional Profile System. Washington, DC, Association of American Medical Colleges. 1989.

AAMC Report on American Medical Education: Institutions, Characteristics and Programs. Washington, DC, Association of American Medical Colleges, 1989.

AAMC Report on Medical School Applicants: Trends 1981–1988 Washington, DC, Association of American Medical Colleges, 1989.

AFCR Newsletter 1989:1(2). Washington, DC, American Federation of Clinical Research.

AMA Physician Characteristics and Distribution in the United States. Chicago, American Medical Association, 1990.

AMA Physician Masterfile. Chicago, American Medical Association.

Andrews E: *A History of Scientific English: The Story of Its Evolution Based on a Study of Biomedical Terminology.* New York, Richard R Smith, 1947.

Applegate WB, Williams ME: Career development in academic medicine. *Am J Med* 1990;88:263–267.

Arias IM: Training basic scientists to bridge the gap between basic science and its application to human disease. *N Engl J Med* 1989;321:972–974.

Bailar JC, Patterson K: Journal peer review: The need for a research agenda. *N Engl J Med* 1985;312:654–657.

Beeson PB: The academic doctor. *Trans Assoc Am Physicians* 1967;80:1–7.

Bernard C: *Claude Bernard and Experimental Medicine.* Cambridge, Mass, Schenkman, 1967.

Bever AT Jr. A quantitative assessment of fundamental and targeted clinical research at NIAMDD. *Perspect Biol Med* 1980;23:S25–S33. (June 1979 symposium on "Clinical Research: Elements for a Prognosis," University of Chicago.)

Beveridge WIB: *The Art of Scientific Investigation.* New York: Vintage Books, undated, 1951 (?).

Bickel J, Morgan TE: Research opportunities for medical students: An approach to the physician-investigator shortage. *J Med Educ* 1980;55:567–573.

Bishop JM: Infuriating tensions: Science and the medical student. *J Med Educ* 1984;59:91–102.

Bulger RJ: *Technology, Bureaucracy, and Healing in America.* Iowa City: University of Iowa Press, 1988.

Burns TW: Physician investigators for academic medicine. *Ann Intern Med* 1984; 101:708–709.

Cannon WB: *The Way of an Investigator: A Scientist's Experiences in Medical Research.* New York, Norton, 1945.

Carpenter CCJ: Today's challenge: Rigorous biomedical science, globally applied. *Trans Assoc Am Physicians* 1988;101:cxx–cxxxiii.

Carter GM, Robyn A, Singer AM: *The Supply of Physician Researchers and Support for Research Training.* Santa Monica, Calif, Rand Institute, 1983.

Carter GM, Winkler JD, Biddle AK: *An Evaluation of the NIH Research Career Development Award.* Santa Monica, Calif, Rand Corporation, 1987.

Castle WB: Functional stresses within fulltime departments of medicine. *Trans Assoc Am Physicians* 1960;73:1–6.

Chapman CB: Medical education: the physician—then, now, and tomorrow, in Vevier C (ed): *Flexner: 75 Years Later.* Lanham, Md, University Press of America, 1987, pp. 47–62.

Cole S, Cole JR, Simon GA: Chance and consensus in peer review. *Science* 1981;214:881–886.

Colloton JW: Academic medicine's changing covenant with society, *Acad Med* 1989;64:55–60.

Comroe JH Jr, Dripps RH: Scientific basis for the support of biomedical science. *Science* 1976;192:105–111.

Corner GW: *A History of the Rockefeller Institute, 1901–1953: Origins and Growth.* New York, Rockefeller Institute Press, 1964.

Cuca JH: NIH grant applications for clinical research: Reasons for poor ratings or disapproval. *Clin Res* 1983;31:453–463.

Daughaday WH: The care and nurture of clinical investigators. *J Lab Clin Med* 1970;75:6–10.

DeKruif PH: *Microbe Hunters.* New York, Blue Ribbon Books, 1926.

DHEW Secretary's Consultants Report: Advancement of Medical Research and Education. Washington, DC, Office of the Secretary, DHEW, 1958.

DHHS Report to President and Congress: Sixth Report on the Status of Health Personnel. DHHS Pub. No. HRS-P-OD-88-1. Washington, DC, DHHS, 1988.

DiBona GF: Whence cometh tomorrow's clinical investigators? *Clin Res* 1979;27: 253–256.

DOE State Higher Education Profiles. Washington, DC, National Center for Educational Statistics, 1988.

DRG Activity Codebook: Organizational Codes and Definitions Used in Extramural Programs. Bethesda, Md, DRG, NIH, 1989.

DRG Ad Hoc Panel on Peer Review: *Sustaining the Quality of Peer Review.* Bethesda, Md, DRG, NIH, 1989.

DRG Competency Roster of NIH Initial Review Groups. Bethesda, Md, DRG, NIH, 1988.

DRG Executive Secretary Responses to 1989 Ad Hoc Panel Report on Peer Review Quality. Bethesda, Md, DRG, NIH, 1990.

DRG Extramural Trends, FY1979–1988. Bethesda, Md, DRG, NIH, 1989.

DRG Extramural Trends, FY1980–1989. Bethesda, Md, DRG, NIH, 1990.

DRG Handbook for Executive Secretaries. Bethesda, Md, DHHS, NIH, DRG, Referral and Review Branch, 1990.

DRG Peer Review Trends: Member Characteristics, 1977–1986 and 1979–89. Bethesda, Md, DRG, NIH, 1986 and 1989, respectively.

DRG Referral Guidelines for Funding Components of PHS. Bethesda, Md, DRG, NIH, 1990.

DRG Referral Guidelines for Initial Review Groups of NIH. Bethesda, Md, DRG, NIH, 1989.

Dubos RJ: Medical utopias. *Daedalus* 1959;88:410–424.

Dubos RJ, Schaedler RW: The effect of the intestinal flora on the growth rate of mice, and on their susceptibility to experimental infections. *J Exp Med* 1960;111: 407–417.

Ebert RH: Medical education at the peak of the era of experimental medicine, *Daedalus,* 115, no. 2; *Proc Am Acad Arts and Sci* 55–81, 1986.

Ebert RH, Ginzberg E: The reform of medical education. *Health Affairs* 1988 (suppl): 5–38.

Eichna LW: Verities in chaos. *Trans Assoc Am Physicians* 1971;84:1–9.

Evered DC, Anderson J, Griggs P, et al: The correlates of research success. *Br Med J* 1987;295:241–246.

Feinstein AR, Koss N, Austin JHN: The changing emphasis in clinical research: I. Topics under investigation. *Ann Intern Med* 1967;66:396–419.

Feinstein AR, Koss N: The changing emphasis in clinical research: II. Sites and sources of the investigations. *Ann Intern Med* 1967;66:420–434.

Finch CA: The shape of clinical investigation. *J Clin Invest* 1961;40:1019–1020.

Fishman AP, Jolly P: Ph.D.s in clinical departments. *Physiologist* 1981;24:17–21.

Flexner A: *Medical Education in the United States and Canada.* New York, Carnegie Foundation for the Advancement of Teaching, 1910.

Fuchs VR: The health sector's share of the gross national product. *Science* 1990;247: 534–538.

Fye, WB: The origin of the full-time faculty system. *JAMA* 1991;265:1555–1562.

Gardner JW: *On Leadership.* New York, Free Press, 1990.

Gasser H: *Medical Research: A Look Ahead.* New York, part of annual Director's Report to Corporation of the Rockefeller Institute for Medical Research, 1951.

Gentile ND, Jolly P, Levey GS, et al: *Research Activity of Full-Time Faculty in Departments of Medicine: Final Report.* Washington, DC, Association of Professors of Medicine and Association of American Medical Colleges, 1987.

Ginzberg E, Dutka AB: *The Financing of Biomedical Research.* Baltimore, Md, Johns Hopkins University Press, 1989.

Glickman RH: The future of the physician scientist. *J Clin Invest* 1985;76:1293–1296.

Goldstein JL: On the origin and prevention of PAIDS. *J Clin Invest* 1986;78:848–854.

Gregg A: *The Furtherance of Medical Research.* New Haven, Yale University Press, 1941.

Handler P, Wyngaarden JB: The bio-medical research training program of Duke University. *J Med Educ* 1961;36:1587–1594.

Harvey A McG: The sorcerer's apprentice. *Trans Assoc Am Physicians* 1968;81:1–6.

Healy B: Innovators for the 21st century: Will we face a crisis in biomedical research brainpower? *N Engl J Med* 1988;319:1058–1064.

Herman SS, Singer AM: Basic scientists in clinical departments of medical schools. *Clin Res* 1986;34:149–158.

Horrobin DF: Peer review: A philosophically faulty concept which is proving disastrous for science. *Behav Brain Sci* 1982;5:217–218.

Ingelfinger FJ: Peer review in biomedical publication. *Am J Med* 1974;56:686–692.

IOM-NAS, *Committee Report on Personnel Needs and Training for Biomedical and Behavioral Research.* Washington, DC, National Academy of Sciences Press, 1985.

IOM Committee Report: A Healthy NIH Intramural Program: Structural Change or Administrative Remedies? Washington, DC, National Academy of Sciences, 1988a.

IOM Committee Report: Resources for Clinical Investigation. Washington, DC, National Academy of Sciences, 1988b.

IOM Report on Research Funding: A Strategy to Restore Balance, Washington, DC, National Academy Press, 1990.

Jolly P, Taksel L, Beran R: U.S. medical school finances. *JAMA* 1988;260:1077–1085.

Jonas HS, Etzel SI: Undergraduate medical education. *JAMA* 1988;260:1063–1071.

Jonas HS, Etzel SI, Barzansky B: Undergraduate medical education. *JAMA* 1989; 262:1011–1019.

Kelch RP, Novello AC: Training pediatric scientists. *Pediatr Res* 1989;25:1–5.

Kelley WN: Are we about to enter the golden era of clinical investigation? *J Lab Clin Med* 1988;111:365–370.

Kennedy TJ Jr: The rising cost of NIH-funded biomedical research. *Acad Med* 1990;2: 63–73.

Kidd, CV: Basic research—description versus definition. *Science* 1959;129:368–371.

Kipnis DM: Clinical biomedical research and training: A challenge for the medical sub-specialties. *J Lab Clin Med* 1979;93:1–5.

Kipnis DM: Biomedical research: A future challenge for clinical departments. *Trans Assoc Am Physicians.* 1983;96:80–87.

Kohler RE Jr: The enzyme theory and the origin of biochemistry. *Isis* 1973;64:181–196.

Kredich NM: Medical research training program, in Gifford JF Jr (ed): *Undergraduate Medical Education and the Elective System.* Durham, NC, Duke University Press, 1978, pp. 139–142.

Kunkel HG: The training of the clinical investigator. *J Clin Invest* 1962;41:1334–1336.

Lederberg J: Cycles and fashions in biomedical research, in Bowers JZ (ed): *Academic Medicine: Present and Future,* North Tarryton, NY, Rockefeller Archive Center, 1982, pp. 202–215.

Lederman LM: Science: The end of the frontier? *Science* 1991(*suppl*):251.

Lehotay DC, Dugas M, Levey GS: A program for training physician-investigators. *J Med Educ* 1982;57:602–608.

Levey GS, Lehotay DC, Dugas M: The development of a physician-investigator training program. *N Engl J Med* 1981;305:887–889.

Lewis T: Clinical science [Harveian Oration, Royal College of Physicians]. *Br Med J* 1933;2:717–722.

Lipsett MB: The optimal use of Ph.D.s in clinical research, in Young FE (ed): *Clinical Investigations in the 1980's.* Washington, DC, Institute of Medicine, NAS, 1981, pp. F-1 to F-7.

Littlefield JW: The need to promote careers that combine research and clinical care. *J Med Educ* 1986;61:785–789.

Lock S: *A Difficult Balance: Editorial Peer Review in Medicine*, London, Nuffield Provincial Hospitals Trust, 1985.

Luft R, Loew H: Excellence and creativity in science. *Clin Res* 1980;28:329–333.

Macy Foundation Report: Clinical Education and the Doctor of Tomorrow. New York, New York Academy of Medicine, 1989.

Merton RK: Basic research and its potentials of relevance. *Mt. Sinai J Med* 1985;52:679–684.

Movsesian MA: Effect on physician-scientists of the low funding rate of NIH grant applications. *N Engl J Med* 1990;322:1602–1604.

Narin F: *Concordance Between Subjective and Bibliometric Indicators of the Nature and Quality of Performed Biomedical Research.* Washington, DC, DHHS, 1983.

NAS-IOM Forum on Supporting Biomedical Research: Near-Term Problems and Options for Action. Washington, DC, National Academy of Sciences, 1990.

NRC-IOM Report on Personnel Needs: Biomedical and Behavioral Research Scientists: Their Training and Supply Washington, DC, National Academy Press, 1989.

Nathan DG: Funding subspecialty training for clinical investigators. *N Engl J Med* 1987;316:1020–1022.

NIH Advisory Committee: Authority, Structure, Function, Members. Bethesda, Md, NIH Director's Office, committee management staff, 1989.

NIH Advisory Committee: Strengthening the Scientific Review Procedures of the NIH Intramural Research Program. Bethesda, Md, Acting Director, NIH, 1990.

NIH Almanac, NIH Pub. 88-5. Bethesda, Md. NIH, 1988.

NIH Clinical Center Review—1985. (chairman: DW Seldin). An in-house staff-written report, September 1985.

NIH Data Book: Bethesda, Md, NIH, 1989 and 1990.

NIH Peer Review Committee Report, Bethesda, MD, NIH, 1988.

NIH Task Force: Review of the NIH Biomedical Research Training Programs, Bethesda, Md, NIH Director's Office, 1989.

NSF: *Characteristics of Doctoral Scientists and Engineers in the United States, 1987. Pub. No. 88-331.* Washington, DC, National Science Foundation, 1988.

Osmond DH: Malice's Wonderland: Research funding and peer review. *J Neurobiol* 1983;14:95–112.

Palca J: Hard times at the NIH. *Science* 1989;246:988–990.

Powledge TM: Fredrickson D: Spending Hughes' legacy. *The Scientist* 1987;1(5):16–17.

President's Biomedical Research Panel Report (chairman: L Thomas). Washington, DC, DHEW, 1976.

Rogers DE: Where have we been? Where are we going? *Daedalus,* 115, no. 2; *Proc Am Acad Arts and Sci* 209–229, 1986 (Spring).

Ross RS: Boundaries of the GCRC in an academic medical center. *Clin Res* 1985;33:105–110.

Ross RS, Johns ME: Changing environment and the academic medical center: The Johns Hopkins School of Medicine. *Acad Med* 1989;64:1–6.

Scheirer MA, Garringer T: *Study of Mail versus Committee Review* Bethesda, Md, NIH Office of the Director, 1990.

Schofield JR: *New and Expanded Medical Schools, Mid-Century to the 1980's.* San Francisco, Jossey-Bass, 1984.

Seldin DW: Some reflections on the role of basic research and service in clinical departments. *J Clin Invest* 1966;45:976–979.

Sherman CR: *Summary of the FY 1987 NIH and ADAMHA Research Support to U.S. Medical Schools,* 1989. An in-house report to the NIH director.

Smith LH Jr: Presidential address. *Trans Assoc Am Physicians* 1976;89:1–9.

Snow CP: *Science and Government.* The 1960 Godkin Lectures on the Essentials of Free Government and the Duties of the Citizen. Cambridge, Mass, Harvard University Press, 1961.

Stossel TP: Reviewer status and review quality: Experience of the *Journal of Clinical Investigation. N Engl J Med* 1985;312:658–659.

Strauss MB: Of medicine, men, and molecules: Wedlock or divorce? *Medicine* 1964;43:619–624.

Strickland SP: *Politics, Science, and Dread Disease.* Cambridge, Mass, Harvard University Press, 1972.

Taksel L, Jolly P, Beran R: U.S. medical school finances. *JAMA* 1989;262:1020–1028.

Thier SO: Clinical investigation in the 1980's: Perspective from the medical schools. *Clin Res* 1980;28:248–251.

Thomas L: Basic science and American business. *Bull NY Acad Med* 1981;57:493–502.

Tobias S: *They're Not Dumb, They're Different.* Tucson, Ariz, Research Corp, 1990.

Wakeford R, Evered D, Lyon J, et al: Where do medically qualified researchers come from? *Lancet* 1985;2:262–265.

Weatherall DJ: *The New Genetics and Clinical Practice.* London, Nuffield Provincial Hospitals Trust, 1982.

Wood WB Jr: Calling Mephistopheles. *Trans Assoc Am Physicians* 1963;76:1–7.

Wyngaarden JB: The clinical investigator as an endangered species. *Trans Assoc Am Physicians* 1979;92:1–15.

Wyngaarden JB: The NIH in its centennial year. *Science* 1987;237:869–874.

Young FE: Introduction of the student physician to research, in Young FE (ed): *Clinical Investigations in the 1980's.* Washington, DC, Institute of Medicine, NAS, 1981, pp. H-1 to H-9.

Index

↑ training of MA + PhD
1960's, 70's + 80's

↑ quality of scientists

↑ # of quality research
application

↑ # Tenured professors
and ongoing projects
devouring funds.

use of MD who is
very young + inexperienced
in research c̄ lots of
experience. This may be
bad but c̄ Greater clinical
experience more i.mpt.

Funds ↑ but cost
of administering projects
also ↑.

Want quick FDA
approval of drugs.

Want Exploratory research
& new discoveries to
be quickly translated
into products, tested
for safety & efficacy
& to the market at
a reasonable price.

Problem

Our present pipeline of R+D is slow and expensive, limiting development of availability of new products. How can we improve availability of new biomedical products.

Background

Complex process of research of biomedical activity development into new products compenses of new to old and test for safety + efficacy,

R&D pipeline is long, expensive + chaotic. Extremely competitive, paper intensive + ↑ cost of administering.

Want a system quicker, less expensive + less paper intensive.

- Budget limitation
- Competition ↑ 2° ↑ # of researchers
- ↑ cost of administration
- ↓ # grants

Protect the public. Limit ineffective, limit harmful, ↑ availability of effective ↓ cost.